Built By History

By

Paul Leonard

Built by History

A personal story of building strength and power through applying the lessons of established strength stars

by Paul Leonard, and Sascha Schnackenberg

Illustration by Miloš Čkonjović

Table of Contents

Forward

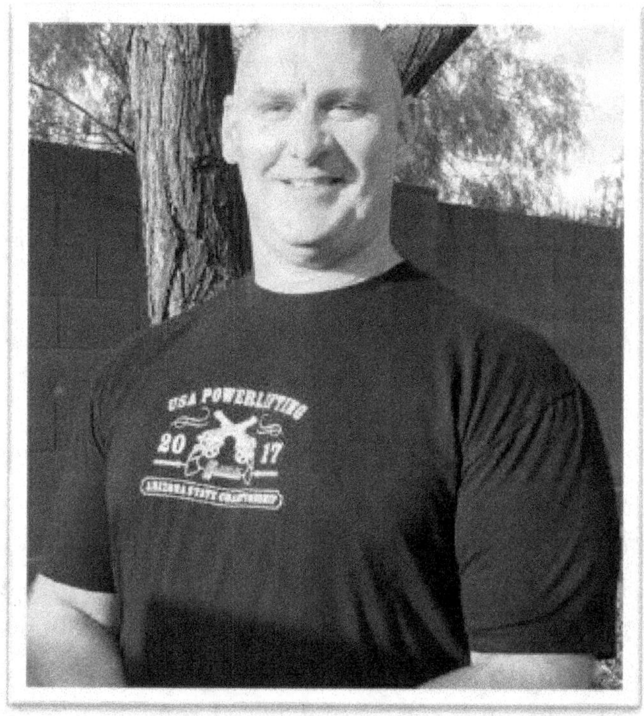

This book is dedicated to anyone who found themselves in a weight room or gym. You are my brothers and sisters.

I have always loved to read about subject I am interested in. To me, the ability to read is like a super power. As soon as I became interested in strength training and powerlifting, I focused my avaricious appetite for knowledge on those subjects. I grew up with the muscle magazines of the day such **as Ironman, Powerlifting USA, Muscle and Fitness, Muscular Development and MuscleMag International**. I read everything I could get my hands on written by Dr. Ken Leistner, Bradley Steiner, Fred Hatfield, Peary Rader, Bill Starr, and Louie Simmons. I began collecting all of the magazines of the day, as well as any books about strength training.

In the late 1990s, once I totaled elite in powerlifting, I felt I had earned the right to author articles for Powerlifting USA Magazine and later Mark Bell's Power Magazine. With the advent of the internet, I wrote for Bodybuilding.com as well as Josh Bryant's website. I was contacted by Sascha Schnackenberg and I began to create content for his website,

Neckberg.com. Sascha has been an ally in creating a site that provides great information, with respect to physical culture's history, about how to train for strength, muscular gains, and bodybuilding success.

I write because I remember what it is like to seek information and how I felt when I discovered the knowledge I was looking for or just became inspired by another's successful iron journey. I have received nothing but positive feedback from my writing and I will always write as it long as it helps just one person. This book is my first, but I intend to write more as I enter my fourth decade of strength training and self discovery through determining my weaknesses and bettering myself every chance I can in the gym. I hope that you the reader get a fraction of the joy, inspiration and knowledge that I have gained in pursuing and sharing my love for physical culture. These are my stories and I am sticking to them.

The Beginning - Mike Lambert's and Peary Rader's Publication

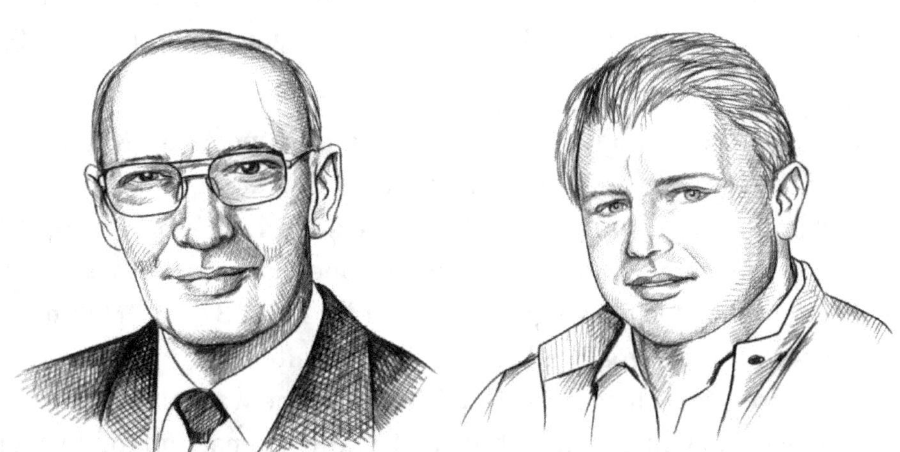

PEARY RADER AND MIKE LAMBERT

Mike Lambert was the creator and publisher of Powerlifting USA Magazine from 1977 to 2012. The magazine was the objective representation of all the different factions and personalities that made up the sport and culture of Powerlifting. During Powerlifting USA's 35 year run it saw other magazines in the U.S. cover the sport of Powerlifting but none of them could claim to be the documented heart and soul of the sport like Mr. Lambert's periodical. To this day, I marvel at finding rare old Powerlifting footage on YouTube that I had only read about, usually in Mike Lambert's words, that confirm Mike's account that the lift was a great lift according to the standards of judging. I have never seen a famous lift which was executed any differently than Mike described in detail.

Mike Lambert was also an amazing photographer as he must have taken over a million Powerlifting pictures in his time as the publisher, all of Powerlifting's superstars and record performers at all the high level meets in the United States as well as abroad. For proof of this concept, Mike published my Bruce Grieg deadlift workout of the month in 2008, but he used a picture he snapped of me pulling the heaviest deadlift in my weight class at the 2003 APF Senior Nationals at Universal Studios.

Despite the proliferation of federations that Powerlifting splintered off into in the 1990s, Mike gave proportionate coverage to every legitimate federation.

Each magazine would have lifter profiles, reports on National or world level meets, a workout of the month, and other interesting and important content. Each issue had a top 100 list of the top 100 squats, benches, deadlifts, and totals done that calendar year in the U.S. for that specific weight class; i.e, 148, 165, 181, etc. Making the list was a huge goal and the list would often adorn the walls of hardcore gyms all over the U.S. The magazine was initially on a 5"X 7" black and white format, then an 8" X 11" format and finally went color in the early 1980s. At the height of Powerlifting's popularity in the late 80s, the magazine offered a companion publication called Power hotline which was released every two weeks for those that could not wait for a once a month injection of knowledge and inspiration. The back half of the magazine was contest results from any sanctioned meet that was submitted to the magazine.

The authors who were a constant source of inspiration and information were Louie Simmons,

Dr Ken Leistner, Marty Gallagher, and contest reporting and profiles by Herb

Glossenbrenner. Once I became a subscriber in 1986, you could mark the first of the month, unless it was a Sunday, as the day that each new magazine arrived in your mailbox. It was not easy to find PLUSA at newsstands in Massachusetts, but once I moved to California in 1991 it was far easier. By the late 90s the magazine was sold at Borders and you were able to find it far easier.

Once I had totaled elite myself I felt I was worthy to give back to the sport by having my writing published in PLUSA. My articles on training partners Art La Bare and Josh Bryant were published in the late 90s to praise from many, to include the GOAT Ed Coan. I have also had articles published on Mike Martin, Patrick Holloway, Mike Tuchscherer, and Bruce Greig.

I met Mike Lambert on a few occasions and he was a very polite and professional individual whom you could tell loved Powerlifting like few others have ever done. His magazine was a labor of love, and it premiered within ten years of the sport of Powerlifting having it's first sanctioned meets, including the Senior nationals and World meets of the early 1970s. Mike always took the high road, never took sides openly with any faction, and only sought to grow and represent the sport of Powerlifting in the most positive light possible. Anyone involved in strength sports today could learn a lot from Mike's lead and dedication to the sport he loves and helped to grow.

Peary Rader: The Most Influential Person of Physical Culture of All time

The role that Peary Rader has played in the establishment of physical culture can not be understated. The founder and editor of Ironman Magazine provided a trusted platform in his periodical that presented timeless training and nutrition information. The boldest move that Peary made in publishing was placing the statement "The Quality Magazine For All Men Interested in Physical Superiority" under the title of Ironman on every cover through out the 1970s. This was no audacious claim, this was a factual statement that has stood the test of time. The strength and bodybuilding legends who were made famous when the pages of Ironman documented their prowess have had indelible impact on physical culture. Before Peary was a publisher he was a man who sought to improve his physical condition.

Peary's Training Philosophy

A YouTube video by the creator Golden Era Bookworm that was released in April 2018 synopsized Peary's training philosophy as detailed in the classic 1947 Your Physique Magazine. Peary believed that a man should train 2 to 3 times per week, with the primary focus being on the breathing squat. A person should train heavy and employ progressive overload by increasing either the weight on the bar or the repetitions done with the weight every time you train. Rader described in his article that 20 repetition squats are brutally hard and can be a mental challenge. To keep from going stale, Peary said a lifter could do one all out set of 20 repetitions, then next workout he could do three sets of ten repetitions and finally the next workout the lifter could do two sets of 15 reps. Peary detailed how alternating your squat repetitions every workout could help avoid the mental drudgery that can be associated with high repetition squatting.

Peary listed the proper workout for gaining size and strength was to do the following exercises:

1. The breathing squat

2. Pullovers for 20 repetitions

3. Military Press for 10 to 12 repetitions

4. Barbell curls/or chin up for 10 to 12 repetitions

5. Bench press/ or dips for 10 to 12 repetitions

6. Bent over Barbell rows for 10 to 12 repetitions

7. Sit ups or leg raises for 10 to 12 repetitions

Peary published an article he wrote in Ironman called combining the 1 1/2 system and rest pause training as being the optimum way to build strength and concurrent size – as opposed to just pumping the muscles up, congesting the muscle with light weights and high repetitions. Peary went into detail with how he had pumped his arms with blood all week via light weights and high repetitions. The result was an arm that was 1" bigger in a week, but could not lift an additional pound in the curl. Lesson learned all. Rader's words from this article which is almost 50 years old was that heavy weights in training used by a strongman provided him with muscles that "to the touch have amazing power, toughness, and permanency,"when compared to a bodybuilder's muscles.

Peary went on to say that some bodybuilders who build big muscles through pumping light weights are never able to build power to match their bloated appearance if they start training correctly with heavy weights and lower repetitions.

Peary credits the rest pause system he has written about in the past, as having been created by Charles Ross, who based his system on the results of controlled medical experiments in muscle building. Rader describes the rest pause method as superior because it allows the trainee to use heavy weights, conserves energy, promotes proper circulation between repetitions, the muscles are fed during the workout and as a result the trainee feels refreshed following training- not exhausted and needing days to recover.

Peary notes that Bruce Page developed the 1 1/2 system that has been described in Ironman Magazine prior to this important article. The 1 1/2 system makes use to the rebound and short movement principles that according to Rader and Page are: " so helpful in muscle building."

Peary elaborated that the squat was the perfect rest pause exercise for gaining strength and size due to the fact that a lifter could take three to six deep breaths between repetitions of the squat. This pause in between squat repetitions forces blood and oxygen to surge through the body- this is the secret to the significant bodily muscle mass gained from an intense rest pause squat session.

Peary detailed combining the two systems during a bench press workout in great detail, describing how a lifter would bench press a loaded bar for one full repetition the immediately press the weight for a half repetition and immediately re-rack the bar. At that point the lifter would watch a clock, count to ten, or take three deep breaths (all three measures take approximately 10 seconds) and begin his next 1 1/2 repetition and re-rack and pause for 10 seconds- doing this sequence for ten total 1 1/2 repetitions with 10 second pauses between each repetition. Rader said with practice, the lifter will develop a rhythm and his sets will be smooth, efficient and effective.

Rader said eventually a lifter would be able to do multiple rest pause sets with approximately 5 minutes rest between each set due to the fact that heavy weight would be utilized.

Peary's article went on to detail how the curl, the row and the deadlift were perfect exercises for the 1 1/2 rest pause system. Peary said that 6 to 8 exercises per training session provided the best results. Rader surprisingly recommended that either 3 days per week full body training sessions could be used or alternatively the split system could be employed during with three upper body workouts and three lower body workouts were completed on alternate days.

In modern times, **super trainer Josh Bryant** has popularized rest pause sets while training the all time world record holder in the bench, **Julius Maddox as well as two other 700lb raw benchers.**

Diet and lifestyle factors Peary Rader espoused

Peary was a man of faith who was no bible thumper, but he did express that a man wishing to build his body needed to abstain from smoking or drinking, while making sure to obtain 8 to 10 hours per night of sleep.

The cornerstone of Peary Rader's gaining program was the drinking of at least two quarts of milk per day. In addition to eating a whole food diet of meat and potatoes, Peary wrote at length about the power of milk-authoring a piece called Milk- Master Bodybuilder. Peary made the influential statement that drinking milk was as important as squats for a man wanting to gain size and strength. Peary described how milk is the perfect food because it contains all the elements in the correct proportion to promote growth. Milk is not a man made food, it is a wonder of nature that can always be used in it's natural state without any special preparation. "Nothing short of miracles have been noted when milk was used as a bodybuilder and weight gainer," stated Peary in Your Physique Magazine. As for your writer I was sold on milk when I began training and by the time I left college, I had squatted 315 for 20 repetitions as well as 615 for 1 in a Powerlifting contest by the age of 22. I am 6'2" and I gained 60 lbs of solid body weight on a heavy milk diet.

Peary the Publisher

Peary began publishing Ironman in 1936 and continued to do so until 1986. The magazine continued to be published after being sold to John Balik, who published quality information until he sold the magazine approximately 5 years ago. Ironman Magazine today is the antithesis of the quality product established by Peary and his wife, Mabel Rader. Peary produced such a quality product he created a legacy and outlasted over 100 Physical Culture magazines that were produced in the U.S. during the time period in which he published Ironman. When the esteemed Mike Lambert stopped publishing Powerlifting USA Magazine in 2012 after 35 years, he proudly posted on his Website that achieving 75% of the longevity of his idol Peary Rader has been a dream come true.

Milo Magazine, which was the closest in content and quality to Ironman, launched 6 years after Rader left the helm of his magazine. Milo had a 25 year run and employed former Ironman writers such as Dr Ken Leistner, Anthony Ditillo, Bruce Wilhelm, and Bradley Steiner. All of these strength writers had different training methodologies, but they all stressed the fundamentals; working as hard as possible, progressive overload, proper rest, and sensible dietary guidelines.

Peary played no favorites as he published content on the top bodybuilders, powerlifters, weight lifters, and athletes who attributed weight training/physical culture for their success. Mr. Rader was a judge at the 1972 Senior National Powerlifting Championships in Denver, Colorado. Following the amazing performance of Jon Cole at that meet, Ironman Magazine published a detailed profile of Jon Cole in 1973 acknowledging that he was the strongest man in the world at that time. Peary helped promote the burgeoning sport of Powerlifting by judging at high level meets to ensure that the athletes were legitimately judged.

Eric Fiorillo and Zach Even Esch have referenced Peary's Ironman on numerous podcasts as being the standard for a half of century with the best information regarding physical culture. Today Josh Bryant, myself, and many others have found their foundation of success in the iron game to be entirely based upon the teachings and content created by Peary Rader, a true physical cultural phenomenon.

Powerlifters, who influenced me

Roger Estep – Powerlifting Immortal

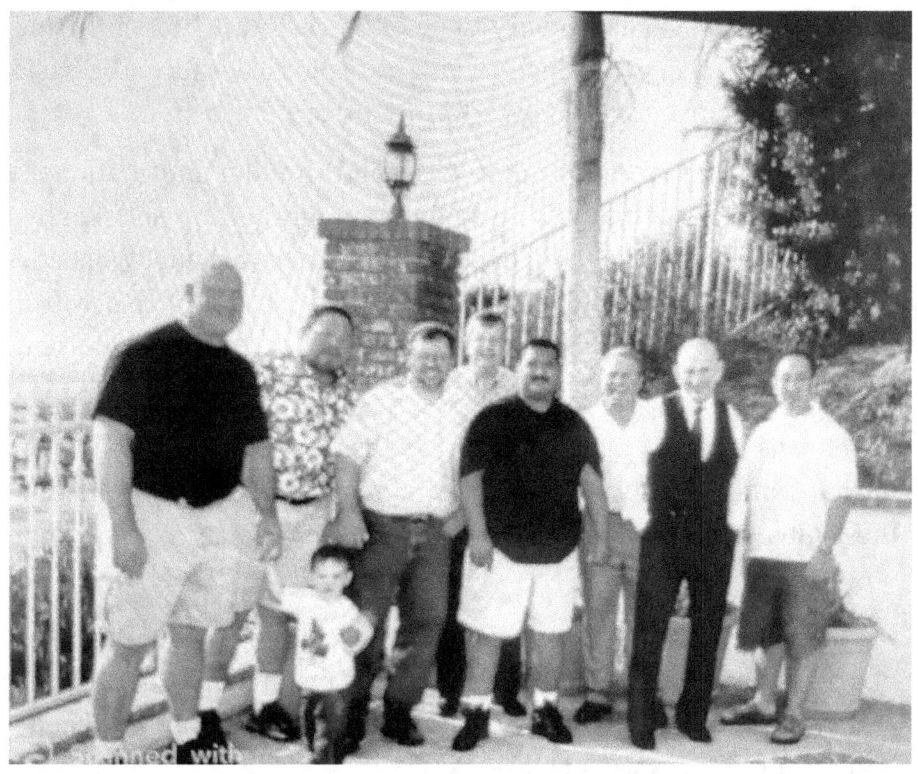

Left to right: Paul Leonard, Lou Leonard, Gary Garcia, ?, Terry McCormick, Manny Sanchez,

*Denny Thompson, **Roger Estep**, Jeff Acura*

I am fortunate to have met and known Roger Estep personally the last ten years of his life. I grew up seeing pictures of Roger in Muscle and Fitness magazine when he was training as a power bodybuilder and contemplating entering physique contests.

Roger sported such a dense physique by the mid 1980s that it was inspirational to look at his images. By 1986, I had discovered Powerlifting USA magazine and began reading Roger's advice column which was very helpful.

In 1988, after I traveled to and came in 2nd at the ADFPA Eastern USA Open in

Gaithersburg, Maryland, at training partner at my gym named Dennis Coholan gave me every issue of Powerlifting USA magazine which had been in print since 1977. These old issues form the basis of my Instagram account, Powerlifting History Illustrated.

These old issues were a goldmine of solid training information as well as the basis of many of my training programs and philosophy. Roger Estep was a huge influence on me with his original Westside Barbell training routine, his great lifts, and his out of this world physique. Everything a young strength athlete wants to be and achieve.

Roger was on the cover of numerous issues, lifting and again in posing trunks once showing what a powerful physique he had. In the 1980s, Roger had a question and answer column in PLUSA that was very helpful.

During the 1980s, Roger was under contract to Joe Weider and his out of this world physique was featured prominently in Muscle and Fitness Magazine, a publication that at one time reached millions of readers world wide.

Roger had an impressive scrap book of memories that he maintained into his last days on earth. He has the letter he received from the Cincinnati Reds Major League Baseball team which was a contract for his skills. The Reds were one of the premier teams in all of baseball during the 1970s, so that will show you the type of athletic ability Roger had. Roger was a terror on the softball fields of Orange County after he stopped training for competition in the lifting sports. A late 1980s PLUSA had a photograph of Roger through during an at bat that displayed incredible form. Readers may not realize this but softball was big in America in the late 1970s into the 1980s, with professional barnstorming teams and television coverage.

In Roger's scrap book was a letter signed by Joe Weider promising a 100,000 per year salary if Roger became a professional bodybuilder. There was a picture in Roger's house signed by multiple time Mr. Olympia winner Frank Zane that was signed to the best built powerlifter in the world. High praise from the best built man of the late 1970s.

Roger was a Nuclear physicist, who owned the California Medical Imaging Registry of Orange, California. Roger's house was beautiful on a steep hillside over looking much of Orange County. You could see the beach from his house, approximately 30 miles away. Roger was extremely financially successful and he shared his wealth with his friends.

In 2002, Roger's health was failing so I posted on the popular powerlifting forum, Go Heavy, that Roger would love to hear from old friends and competitors. The outpouring of emotion and support from so many strength stars of the 1970s was impressive.

This posting also led to Roger re-kindling an old relationship that led to his marriage the following year!

Roger passed away on June 23, 2005, at the age of 57 from complications of treatment for glioblastoma. There was some speculation that this type of cancer could be caused by Roger's work and subsequent exposure to nuclear material.

Roger was married and had 4 step daughters at the time of his premature demise. He has recently been remembered as the platform monster he was by the immortal Louie Simmons in his book the Iron Samurai.

I highly recommend this book! Louie has always said he was jealous that Roger got to leave Ohio and train with the original Westside Barbell Culver City legends. Like Roger, I myself was better for moving to California to pursue my powerlifting dreams.

Bill Kazmaier – The World's Strongest Man

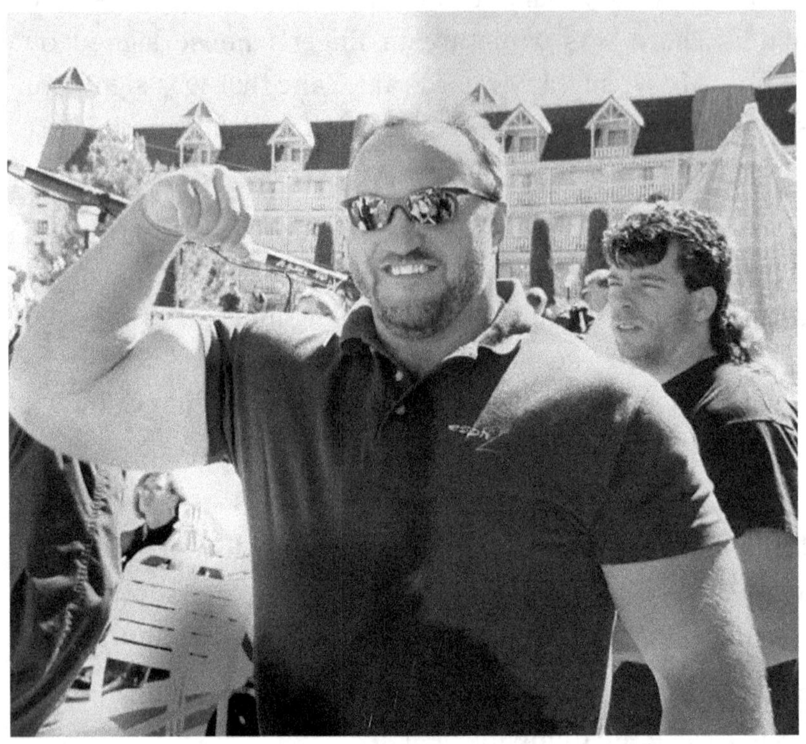

The Kaz has graced us with a great deal of social media information such as YouTube videos with Josh Bryant, many of his European seminars appear online, as well as his own Instagram postings. Kaz's induction speech into the Arnold a Sports Hall of Fame is must see viewing. Despite these gems online, there is nothing like listening to the self proclaimed Strongest man who ever lived in person. That quote from Kaz at the 1982 WSM Contest to a British broadcaster was not said boastfully, just factually. Kaz today in person is a very humble and captivating speaker.

The first thing you realize when you are in Kaz's presence is that he is very athletic in appearance despite being over 60 years of age. Kaz is also still fucking huge. There is no other way to say it. I myself had only met Kaz once before at the 1997 WSM in Las Vegas and I was impressed with him then, but even more so now, almost 20 years later.

Kaz described his philosophy in lifting as being heavily influenced by Iron Icon **Bill Pearl**, who authored the **Keys to the Inner Universe**, a very influential book for Kaz. Kaz played football in high school, specifically nose guard and fullback, graduating at 222 lbs after also competing in the shot put as well as the 100 meter dash. Kaz said that when he was 215lbs in high school he could press his body weight for a set of 5.

Kaz also wrestled in high school and entered the University of Wisconsin after graduation. Kaz dropped out of school and began his Powerlifting odyssey at the Madison YMCA. Kaz fondly recalled his early influences from the YMCA, specifically Bob Lowrie, Mike Morgan, and his best partner Steve Disalvo.

Kaz recalled that he was benching 300 initially after entering college but within a matter of months he was benching 400.

The first time Bill deadlifted was his first day of college when he pulled 600. Genetics anyone?

Despite obvious physical gifts, Bill came from what I would describe as an abusive household. Bill did not describe his relationship with his father as abusive, but I would after hearing about it. Bill said that his father often described him as horse shot and detailed a story of how his father once hit him with a brick in the back from a distance. These stories really put into perspective Kaz's accomplishments now that it is public knowledge that Kaz had anything but a supportive father-son relationship.

Bill stated that he developed his incredible work ethic at an early age because he worked for a tree surgeon during which he had to cut and haul trees from beside a lake up to a work truck.

Kaz's work ethic immediately endeared him to California Powerlifters such as Joe Free and Bud Ravenscroft. Kaz described that once in California **he would often do 7 sets of 7 reps for**

many of his exercises, intensely telling the seminar that by set 4 or 5 he would be "rolling." Kaz who held the world record Powerlifting total for almost the entire decade of the 80s, had competitive bests of 925 661 837 2425. Kaz fondly recalled some of his gym repetition personal records such as deadlifting 650 for 10, cheat curling 315 for 15 with lots of back heave, and dumbbell pressing 156lb dumbbells for a set of 10.

Kaz told the audience about his usual bench press workout which included 550 for 5 sets of 5 with a down-set of 430lbs for 30 reps, not locking out the reps because he always trained triceps the day after bench pressing. Kaz proudly described that he would "smash" 35 to 47 work sets for his lats while occasionally supersetting rear delt work between. **Kaz had a preference for higher reps and this continued into his retirement** from contests when Kaz described that he would powerbuild his delts by seated pressing the 100s for 38 reps when he was in his late 40s.

Kaz broke down his philosophy for training each of the power lifts, beginning with the squat. Kaz was influenced in how he trained the squat by Powerlifting legends Dave Shaw and Bruce Randall. Kaz stated that in 1979 he was correctly fitted for his first TMJ splint and as a result he was able to correctly harness the power of his teeth, the most important of the 12 neurosystems of the body. **Kaz also used custom made Addidas power boots which kept his knee inline with his ankle**. At his peak, Kaz squatted 900 for 3 in the gym as he tried to become the first powerlifter to officially squat 1000lbs. Kaz was never able to squat a grand in a meet but he did complete squatting movements in Strongman contests that were more than half a ton.

Kaz described his mental attitude towards squatting as "loathing the weights", getting agitated before a heavy set and always striving to increase his pain tolerance. Kaz spoke often about meditation and visualization. For those of us who had Kaz's training manuals when in college we recall they were signed with the phrase "conceive, believe, achieve." Kaz said that he would envision a red light and a green light which was the signal his brain was receiving from a heavy weight. Kaz believed he was in such control of his mind that he could re-wire his mind to over ride the red light and see green. "When others quit, hit the gas."

Kaz referred to his famous traps as Mt Fugi and Mt Kilamangaro, stating that he trained them heavy as possible with sets of shrugs such as 650 lbs for 50! Kaz said he believed that training should focus on doing as much base work as possible because the bigger the base the higher the pyramid can rise. Kaz spoke of of completing 12 weeks cycles with high reps for all 3 of the lifts. Kaz talked of cycling his poundages from 70 percent to 100 percent during the 12 week cycle. Kaz remarked that he would set short term and long term goals in regards to a workout, a week of workouts, and for months at a time. Kaz said he was analytical and would make minor adjustments to each workout. Kaz knew that he could bench 50 lbs more than his top triple from training.

He described that he could not bench 135 the day after heavy squats. This was the result of the cramming his ridiculously jacked 340lb body under the standard squat bar. Kaz said when he benched he would maintain a 90 degree angle when the bar was on his chest. **Kaz said if this angle was not present then all the stress would be on the pec.** Kaz said that during his peak years benching he was hard, fast and reckless when he benched as well as when he lowered the bar. Kaz stressed training your delts hard for bench press success, stating that the range of motion for delts is short and demonstrated some side and front raises. "You have to make delts burn to grow."

For tricep strength Kaz stated he preferred decline tricep presses for 10 to 15 reps. Kaz spoke of warming up to deadlift heavy with lighter, high bar style squats. "You should look like a sewing machine, going straight up and down, doing non-lock squats. Kaz said that the body really has to be pushed because the body can take "a lot of weight." Not to think that this was your average light day, Kaz cited sets of over 600lbs for 15 reps to build his leg drive for the deadlift. Squatting legend Marvin Phillips taught Kaz these non lock squats and a as a result he built world class hip flexor strength like that mentor.

Kaz stated he utilized very heavy partial squats leading into a meet, lifting the bar concentrically from pins in the power rack working with 100lbs over his max. Kaz said he also utilized rack deadlifts with very heavy weights. **Kaz remarked that deadlift god John Kuc once told Kaz he did 150 sets of upper back per week.** No wonder he pulled 870 at

242. **"When you pull a deadlift, push your feet through the floor," was Kaz's words of wisdom.** To keep the front of his back strong, i.e. his abs, Kaz loved twists on a hyper bench as well as decline sit-ups with a 100lb plate.

Kaz made a very profound statement when asked to discuss why 99.9 percent of most powerlifters will not approach his records.

"Lifters need to get in better shape, they need to lean up, build muscle, dial in their form, and go back to go forward."

Kaz cited Andy Bolton of being the perfect example of a lifter who needs to apply his knowledge. Kaz said that except for squats, the rest between sets should be 1.5 to 2 minutes. Push the volume and amount of work done per work up constantly. Calves, abs, and traps should be trained with high volume and frequency. Kaz did not track workout tonnage, he believed in training hard, fast and intense.

Kaz spoke very highly of many of his contemporaries such as Jon Cole-"probably the best strength athlete ever", OD Wilson-a great guy, and Tom McGlaughlin, who was a genius.

Like most big strong men, Kaz spoke intelligently about food. "The more mass you have, the harder you can contract."

Kaz closed out the seminar with such gems as "Your perception of reality is your reality." "Honestly assess where you are at and where you are going" in your training and competitive career.

My day with Kaz was extremely memorable. In my 50s now, I have been amazed by him since I was a teenager. Getting to know him in person and over lunch that day was a day I learned so much and validated the course I have lived my life as a strength athlete. It was great to see the fellowship which exists between Kaz and modern day strength monster Jerry Pritchett. It gets no better than that Neckberg fans.

Thank you to Kaz and for Jerry Pritchett and his incredible family for making that day a reality.

Anthony Clark – Inventor of the Reverse Grip Benchpress

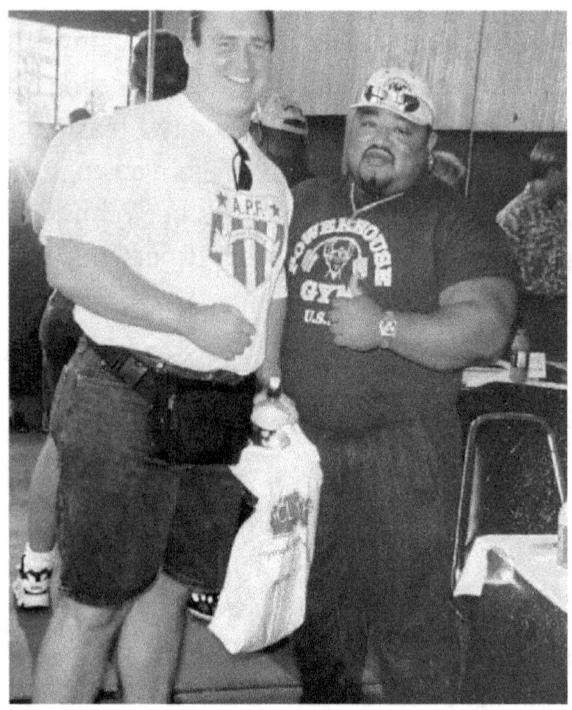

Most people now who know of the late, great Anthony Clark, associate his name with the first assault on the 800lb bench press. For those of us who grew up powerlifting in the 80s, Anthony was a well rounded strength athlete who pushed up the all time total and squat record- as well as performed strength exhibitions that captured the lifting world's attention, such as the December 1990 Powerlifting USA Magazine on which the cover showed Anthony walking with a Subaru Brat like a wheelbarrow!

Anthony's official lifts according to Open Powerlifting,org of a 1031 squat 770 bench press and a 730lb deadlift with an official total of 2531 in multiple ply supportive gear as well as a 1025 squat 750 bench and 744 deadlift with a 2408 total only tell part of his story. Anthony was one of the highest profile powerlifters of his time with sponsorship from a clothing line called Lator, Toka belts, Inzer support gear, and Powerhouse Gym- of which he owned a franchise in the Houston area.

Anthony competed at all the major meets of his era such as the Budweiser World Record Breakers, the Arnold Classic, the WPO, and numerous National and World Championship competitions. Anthony received mainstream media coverage on ESPN when he lofted at the 1988 Hawaiian Open as well as on Powerlifter Video Magazine, and in all the publications of his time that covered strength training such as Muscle and Fitness, Muscular Development, MuscleMag International and numerous cover appearances on Powerlifting USA Magazine.

I first read about Anthony in PLUSA when there was a picture and a report of him winning the 1986 Teenage Nationals with a 611lb bench press and a 1940lb total! I had number copies in my gym of Anthony, particularly the shot from Muscle and Fitness of him close grip incline benching 585!

I first met Anthony at the 1991 Malibu Classic Bench Press and Deadlift meet in Southern California. At this meet Anthony benched 617 and deadlifted 717. I was impressed seeing him in person.

Anthony was still gripping the bench press bar the same way as everyone else, but in 1993 he began competing with a reverse grip in the bench. To see Anthony bench was amazing as he would control a third of a ton in his hand and bring the bar down to his chest under control and then lock it out fully in accordance with the rules. Anthony was heavily scrutinized during his prime- as all ATWR benchers are, but Anthony won the Greatest Bench in America as well as the Arnold Classic Bench Press Championships against the best in the world- breaking the ATWR at least half a dozen times with 735, 744, 751, 766, 770. Anthony took many close tries at 800lbs but was unable to complete this lift in competition.

Next time I met him was in 1997 at the Mr. Olympia Bodybuilding Exposition in Long Beach, California. Anthony looked great, larger than I remembered him from 1991 and he was promoting his various sponsors.

The last time I saw Anthony was at the 2000 WPO Inaugural Meet in Daytona Beach, Florida. In a matter of a few years, Anthony's health had deteriorated since I had last seen him. He was suffering from jaundice and had trouble breathing as he walked.

Anthony had been a world class squatter during his career, setting records in the new IPA

Federation that began in the 90s, with a 1031 effort and a miss with 1100! In the early 90s Anthony had a squatting accident at the huge Texas Grand meet in which he fell underneath 992 lbs but didn't get seriously injured!

Sadly Anthony passed away far too young. He and I shared a mutual friend who said that Anthony actually died of a broken heart because he was in love with a woman who did not treat him well. Anthony had overcome so many things in his life. He was born in the Philippines and immigrated to the U.S. when he was 7 years old. His early days in the U.S. were very hard for him as he was extremely skinny and being in a predominantly white area, he was picked on, bullied and beat up for being different than the other kids in his neighborhood.

Anthony described many times how he resisted the temptation to get involved in drugs and alcohol to escape his reality. Anthony was a man of great faith and often preached that all power comes from God, who had saved Anthony. Anthony began working out at the age of 13, when he weighed 120lbs. At his strongest, Anthony would grow to weigh 325lbs and have 23" arms at a height of 5'7". The first time I saw Anthony in person, I amazed at how dense and thick his musculature and joints were.

At Anthony's peak of popularity, he was filmed pretty extensively, as his lifts were exciting and ground breaking. Texas had a very robust powerlifting culture in the 90s - with many huge meets that

Anthony participated in. Anthony also traveled a great deal and performed in front of many fans. Pictures of Anthony always inspired because he was larger than life and handled amazing weights in training that were forever captured in film. I have seen Ryan Kennelly in person, trained at the same gym as CT Fletcher- but when it comes to arm strength and development no one could match Anthony and his reverse grip power.

Ken Leistner – An Incredible Strength Influence

DR. KEN LEISTNER MENTORING ME PRIOR TO MY FARMERS WALK ATTEMPT IN 2002 AT THE NORTHEAST STRONGMAN

As soon as I became obsessed with powerlifting, I immediately began reading everything I could get my hands on such as Powerlifting USA. Dr Ken Leistner was the training editor for that magazine since its inception in 1977 until 2012 when the magazine ceased production. Dr Ken was a staple in Muscular Development Magazine during the eighties with great articles and pictures of his ridiculously hard training followers such as Kevin Tolbert. With the creation of Milo Magazine in 1993, Dr. Ken was a contributor to that quarterly publication for approximately 25 years as well. Dr Ken wrote a blog for the Powerlifting Support Equipment Company Titan called "History of Powerlifting, Weightlifting, and Strength Training- completing 124 posts from 2014 until the last post which was published 5 days before his sudden death on April 6, 2019. To be honest, I am shocked that there has been no post or written tribute to this great man on the Titan Blog/Website.

Online I was able to locate a very well done tribute piece on a website called Training and

Conditioning. The Generation Iron Website published an awesome tribute to Dr. Ken entitled "Remembering the Influential Strength Coach Dr. Ken Leistner" written by Johnathan Salmon, and published 4 days after Dr Ken's death.

I will write this piece from my heart as I knew Dr Ken personally and I will explain how he influenced me greatly. I love to read about strength training and competitions almost as much as I like to train and compete in them. As soon as I began Powerlifting training and competitions in 1986, I subscribed to _Powerlifting USA Magazine_. Dr. Ken had a monthly column in that magazine that really formed my training philosophy that you must train as hard as humanly possible to make gains in strength and size. Recovery from training was critical in order to avoid overtraining and injury. Dr. Ken was a lifetime educator as well as a health care professional, i.e. a doctor of chiropractic medicine. In the late eighties Dr. Ken was published in Muscular Development Magazine with fantastic pictures accompanying his articles.

In 1988, a very kind and benevolent training partner named Dennis Coholan gave me every PLUSA magazine that had been produced since it's inception in 1977, as well as a binder with the entire collection of the Steel Tip, a newsletter authored by Dr. Ken for 3 years. I would devour these newsletters as well as the PLUSAs, many of which had multiple Dr Ken articles in them. Dr. Ken wrote at least one training article per magazine, but he would also write contest result reports for World Championships or profile various strength personalities. To this day, I still utilize information that I learned from the Dr's writings.

In addition to hammering the point home that hard and brief work, from which you were able to correctly recover, is the key to an increase in the resistance you train with – Dr. Ken provided interesting ideas on odd object lifting and how to make conditioning strength oriented. Many of the Muscular Development articles had awesome photos showing Dr. Ken and his maniacal trainees like Kevin Tolbert lifting kegs, anvils, wooden barrels, I-beams, chains, and even de-fused bombs! Dr. Ken opened my eyes as a teenager to all the various implements and modalities that could be used to strengthen a lifters body and spirit in a motivating and functional way.

In the summer of 1987, I got my first physical labor job, working at the Waltham Engineering Corporation in Waltham, Massachusetts. The company building was a huge turn of the century factory built on the Charles River that was being refurbished for modern office spaces. My assignments involved stripping old tile floors down to the original wood that had become popular again in the eighties. Wearing safety goggles and using a chisel while another co-worker heated the floor up with a torch, I would hammer off the old tile to reveal the wood underneath the ceramic tile material and layer of old tar. This was tedious back breaking work at times – with the only reward being the opportunity to take a wheelbarrow, once loaded with debris, out of the building to a dumpster.

The other college kids who were working this summer job with me avoided any hard work like the plague but I reveled in it, primarily due to my father's work ethic as well as Dr Ken's writings about his family's work ethic, how being an iron worker made him stronger, and how physical labor made you tougher both physically and mentally. I had strained my back in June deadlifting and so for that summer of manual labor, I worked around the deadlifts by doing loading, demolition, and weighted carrying. I had never heard of the concept of GPP, which Louie Simmons talked about over a decade later – but this was exactly what I built then. By the end of the summer, my bench press- which I focused on that summer, was strong enough to win the Massachusetts Teenage American Drug Free Powerlifting Federation State Championship with a 315 at 220lbs. I had put 50 pounds on my bench press since graduating high school the previous year. This was done by doing manual labor from 6 am to 2 pm, then immediately going to the gym after work to train 4 days per week. I learned such discipline as a teenager due to reading about Dr. Ken and other strong men he had worked with or trained over the years.

Fast forward ten years and I was established in a professional career and living in Southern California. Much like many of Dr Ken's stories about his youth, when I was old enough to travel from the east coast to California, I relocated there and did not just visit. I had a great garage gym in Orange County called Yorba Barbell and I began selling a tape of our training in the garage via a message board for powerlifting called Go Heavy. I was contacted by Dr. Ken who wanted to purchase the tape so I sent him one immediately. Dr. Ken wrote about my tape in a 1999 Powerlifting USA article he authored, endorsing the tape. This made sales of the 2 hour VHS tape skyrocket and I was able to buy many more pieces of equipment for the gym, as well as travel to the 1999 IPA World Powerlifting Championships in York, Pennsylvania.

1993 was a great year for strength training enthusiasts, as the great training publication Milo was first published. This quarterly journal contained Dr. Ken's articles as well- with an emphasis on training programs that work to get stronger and bigger. Now serious lifters would get Dr Ken in PLUSA until 2012 and Milo until 2018. Following the cessation of both publications, Dr Ken's writing appeared on the Titan Support Systems Website until 5 days before his passing. Dr. Ken loved and coached football at various levels and his writings about that sport can be found on Helmet Hut. The owner of that site posted a moving tribute about Ken's passing.

There are some great YouTube videos of Dr Ken, including a famous one that is legend in the hard core strength community of Dr. Ken's workout he filmed to be sold to raise charity for a local charity that was important to the Dr. The clip appears on STG Strength and Power's YouTube channel. It was filmed on April 22, 2000. Dr. Ken opens the tape by saying he is making the tape for his family, so that his kids can see how he trained if for some reason he was to drop dead. The tape has to be seen to be believed because he is so strong and appears healthy as any high level strength athlete. I had heard of this tape but did not know I could have purchased it back in the early 2000s – I would have. I had not seen this tape until approximately 2019, at the time the Dr. passed.

Less than two years after the tape was created, I got to first meet Ken at the 2002 Northeast Strongman Showdown, where I competed. Dr. Ken and I met before the competition and he immediately began motivating me and inspiring me to do my best that day in the contested events. The Dr. was extremely motivating in person and he got me plenty fired up to do my best.

Lay the foundation for a powerlifting career with lessons from Dr. Ken:

Dr. Ken practiced what he preached, as evidenced by his YouTube clip. Anyone who can squat over 400 for 20 plus reps is strong as hell. When I was in college, I worked up to a set of 315 for 20 deep reps in the squat. Such offseason work, i.e. when I was not getting ready for meet, really built my muscle mass and mental tenacity.

Dr. Ken stressed balanced training, hitting every muscular structure on your body with a compound exercise. I learned how to stiff leg deadlift from the Dr, as well as how to make sure I train my back of my body was hard as the front, showy muscles.

As for how to grow the biggest arms possible, his advice was to build up to 200 lbs for ten reps in the strict curl. I was never able to do this feat, but I did have 20" arms when I got over 300lbs in bodyweight.

Dr.Ken always wrote with a sense of respect and reverence for the history of Powerlifting and it's founding fathers. I always try to emulate Dr. as I have nothing but positive information to write and share about the greatest strength sport in the world.

Josh Bryant – Trainer of Champions

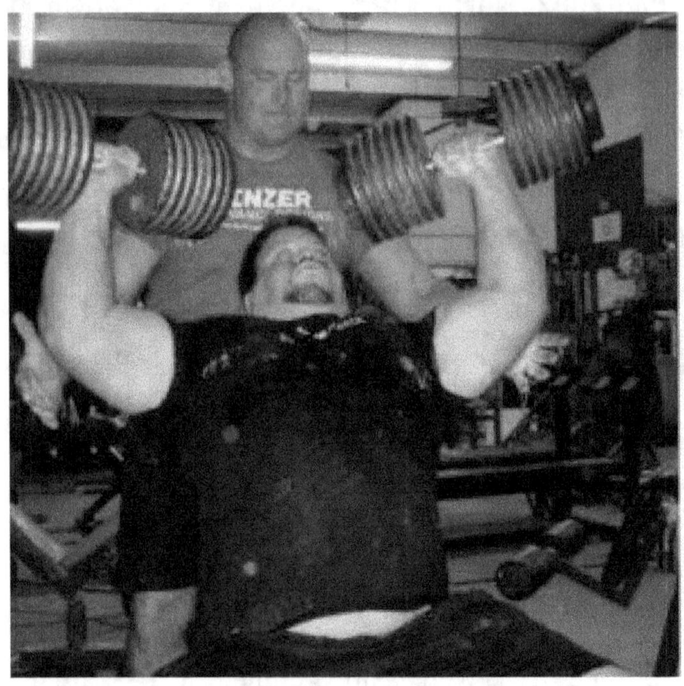

Josh Bryant is the best strength coach in the World, with more world class strength athletes under his current tutelage than any other. Josh currently programs Julius Maddox, Brian Shaw, James Strickland, Jeremy Hoornstra, and Thomas Davis. Josh has worked with Professional Bodybuilders Johnny Jackson and Branch Warren as well as mega bencher Al Davis, Peter Egette, Rob Wilkerson and Chad Wesley Smith.

I am writing this piece during the world wide pandemic that has gyms closed, personal interaction discouraged, and every online trainer in the industry releasing content of how to do body weight exercises. During this time period, Josh has doubled down on his high quality content with YouTube interviews of four time WSM winner Brian Shaw, Bench Legend Jamie Harris, Powerlifting Hall of Fame Member Vince Anello, Strength Coach extraordinaire Bill Gillespie – and these were created and released in one week!

I have known Josh since he was a teenager, albeit one who could bench 500 raw, all while working towards being the world's best three lift powerlifter. Josh rose quickly to become the youngest lifter in the world to bench 600 raw, ultimately ending up with a 620 raw bench, in addition to an official 810 deadlift and a 903 lb squat at the 2003 APF Seniors at Universal Studios Hollywood. Josh won the Atlantis Strongest Man in America Contest in 2005, with an

885 trap bar deadlift, 600lbs raw bench, 445lbs standing press, and a parallel grip pull up with 130 lbs strapped to his body. The head judge of this event was the GOAT, Powerlifter Ed Coan.

After trying his has hand at strongman contests, Josh focused on Bodybuilding style training with allies Brian Dobson, Branch Warren, and Johnny Jackson in Josh's adopted home of Texas. Josh did not enter a bodybuilding contest, but he shaved off some body fat and built up his musculature while giving his joints a break from the heavy pounding he gave them from age 15 to his late 20s.

Josh grew up in the Santa Barbara, California area and was initially a boxer from the Primo

Boxing Gym of Santa Barbara, fighting in some of the roughest barrio boxing gyms in

Oxnard, California. Like most red blooded American males Josh was impressed with Pro Wrestlers at an early age, played high school football, and was an alpha male in an alpha family of his dad, Big Dan Bryant and his younger brother Noah, who was an All American Weight thrower at USC. Josh became best friends with Adam Ben Shea, a Brazilian Jiu Jitsu Blackbelt under the Paragon Jiu Jitsu School. Together they founded Jailhouse Strong, a strength and conditioning business which sells training instruction, programming, administers seminars, and creates written, video and podcast content. Josh's expertise has afforded him a position on the prestigious Elite FTS Staff.

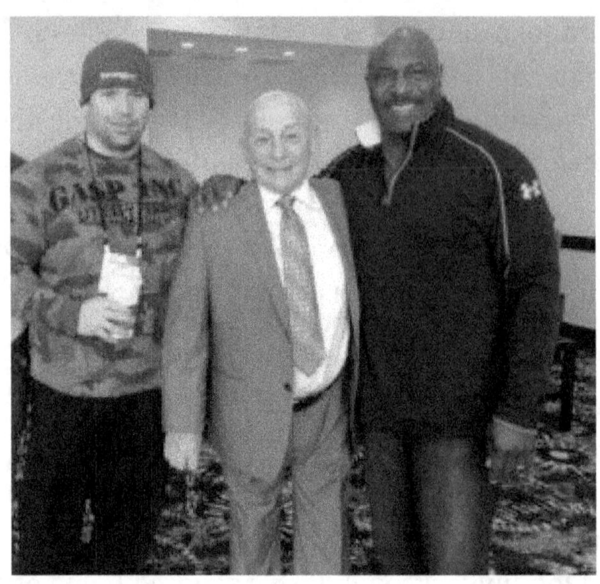

Josh Bryant, Fred Hatfield And Lee Haney

Josh has had many mentors in the strength sports, starting with Steve Holl, George Brink, Ed Coan, Gary Frank, Odd Haugen, Sal Aria, and most of all Fred Hatfield. Josh would drive over 130 miles to my garage gym to squat with me, Art Labare, Gary Hogan, and Gary Garcia beginning in 2000 and continuing this process for years so that he was around driven powerlifters. Josh moved to Baton Rouge, Louisiana to train with Gary Frank when Gary was at his peak, finally settling in the strength rich environment of Dallas/Fort Worth Area.

Josh trains hard to this day, focusing on being gas station ready with resistance training for the whole body, boxing training, sprinting, and conditioning to be ready for whatever challenge life throws his way. I am proud to call Josh a friend, as he is a young man who has lived his competitive and now his professional dreams by creating a business that helps so many, has preserved the concept of physical culture, and sincerely loves the strength sports and allies like Neckberg which keeps the roots of strength alive by sharing the history of what is important.

Fred Hatfield

People I am going to talk with you today about the concept of intensity as it applies to getting stronger. Now, intensity is not the buzz you get in your face from C-4, nor is it the feeling you get when your favorite jam is blasting on the radio. No, intensity is a mathematical factor that will determine how successful you are in achieving your strength and size goals. I have studied the best strength athletes in the world and when I focus on their training, I see more similarities than differences.

When I began my Powerlifting journey in 1986, the great Fred Hatfield, aka Dr Squat, was a world record holder and the powerlifter who wrote the most about the best way to train to get strong. Fred earned a PHD, was the Editor in Chief of Muscle Fitness Magazine and he totaled at the elite level in 5 Powerlifting weight classes from the mid 70s til 1988. He traveled to Russia to learn from their great strength minds, he created a video called Heavy Iron which documented his training theory of compensatory acceleration (This video is free on YouTube.), and he set world records in the squat that can be found online as well as many of his writings. In 1986 Dr Squat shocked the strength world by doing a 1008lb squat at 256 lb body weight at the Hawaii Record Breakers, which was at the time, the greatest meet in the world and televised on ESPN. Fred was 46 when he did this all time world record and looked,bigger than life on the VHS tape of the meet my training partners and I watched on a daily basis. Fast forward to 1993 and I am walking down the Venice Beach Boardwalk when I bump into Fred in person. To say he was small be kind as he was very cordial yet tiny. I became convinced right then and there that this man was a genius because he got such an amazing performance out of such a small, genetically challenged body.

One of the corner stones of Fred's training philosophy is his Russian peak program. The program is a six week peaking cycle that can be used for any lift, but it works very well for the three powerlifts, the squat, bench, and deadlift. The key to the program is the intensity level. Fred learned from his trips to Russia that they key intensity metric is to do the proper amount of volume with 80 percent. Eighty percent is the magic number which will allow a person to gain strength without over training.

Dr Squat's 6 week Russian Peak Program goes as such:

Week 1: Work out # 1 do 6 sets of 2 reps with 80% of your max

Work out # 2 do 6 sets of 3 reps with 80% of your max

Work out #3 do 6 sets of 2 reps with 80% of your max

Week 2: Work out #1 do 6 sets of 2 reps with 80% of max

Work out #2 do 6 sets of 4 reps with 80% of max

Work out #3 do 6 sets of 2 reps with 80% of max

Week 3: Work out #1 do 6 sets of 2 reps with 80% of max

Work out # 2 do 6 sets of 5 reps with 80% of max

Work out # e do 6 sets of 2 reps with 80% of max

Week 4: Work out #1 do 6 sets of 2 reps with 80% of max

Work out # 2 do 6 sets of 6 reps with 80% of max

Work out # 3 do 6 sets of 2 reps with 80% of max

Week 5: Work out #1 do 5 set of 5 reps with 85% of max

Work out #2 do 6 sets of 2 reps with 80% of max

Work out # 3 do 4 sets of 4 reps with 90% of max

Week 6: Work out #1 do 3 sets of 3 reps with 95% of max

Work out # 2 do 6 sets of 2 with 80% of your max

Work out # 3 do 2 sets of 2 reps with 100% of your max

There you have it people, a state of the art Russian strength cycle that drives the correct intensity matched with the correct volume- you end up increasing your work load from 12 reps with 80 percent to 36 reps with 80. You triple your workload in three weeks. The following 3 weeks you decrease the volume and up the intensity to the 85, 90, and 95% - finally peaking by doubling your max in 6 weeks.

I follow this program to this day and I made considerable gains in strength and size with this program throughout my late teens and early 20s.

For more information about Fred Hatfield check out the Jailhouse Strong YouTube content they created with Dr Squat before his recent passing. John Welbourn at Power Athlete has also done podcast work with Dr. Squat that is incredible.

Fred Hatfield truly was a genius and thankfully he shared so much of his knowledge. As most real strong people are never afraid to release their "secrets" because hard work and a laser focus on your goals is no real secret at all-just the truth.

Manfred Hoeberl – The Largest Arms in The World

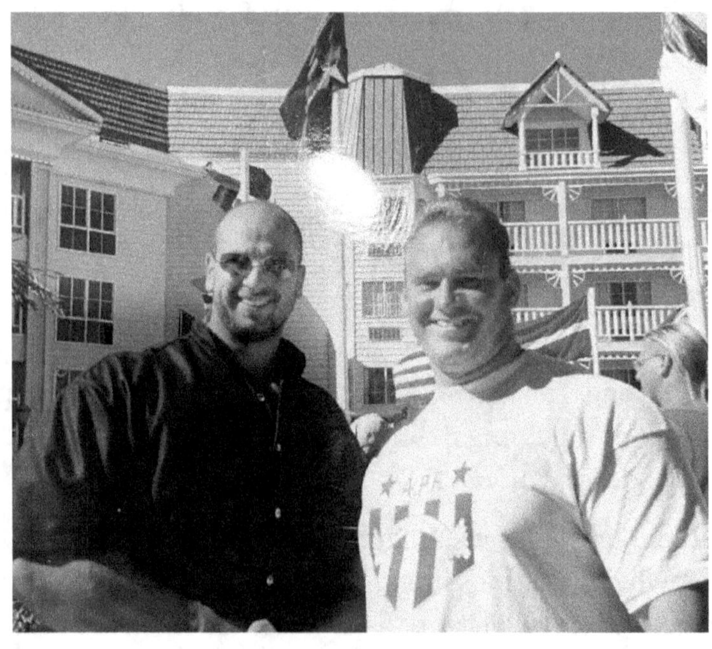

Recently I listened to the excellent podcast that Lawrence Shaleigh did on 90s strongman competitor, Manfred Hoeberl. Manfred literally burst onto the strongman scene by winning the World Muscle Power Championships and almost beating Magnus ver Mangnusson at the 1994 World Strongest Man Contest. Manfred appeared in all the major muscle magazines of that era with his million watt smile and huge muscular physique-complete with what were billed as and appeared to be the largest arms in the world. A popular book was published detailing Manfred's arm training, that is no longer in print.

Just as meteoric as his rise, Manfred's strongman career ended just as abruptly as he rose to fame, Manfred's career was cut short by injuries. Manfred was born on May 12, 1964, and he reached a peak height of 6'4" and 297lbs at his competitive peak. Manfred was born in Graz, Austria the same town that gave the world Arnold

Schwarzenegger. Following his rash of injuries, Manfred's weight dropped to 220lbs.

Manfred Today

Manfred relocated permanently to Dubai in December of 2020. Manfred likes the sunny climate of Dubai and compared the climate to South Africa, where Manfred's strongman career began in the early 1990s. Manfred referenced that his 85 year old mother stays with him for months at a time in Dubai. Manfred said that he is extremely healthy today, his arms are healthy. After recovering from so many health challenges, Manfred developed the philosophy of be happy with what you have. "Live in the moment." "Lifters are never satisfied." Life is so simple said Manfred, seek inner peace and happiness. Manfred spoke so intelligently, it is no surprise that he makes his living being a motivational speaker as well as a mediation instructor.

Manfred's Career as a Strongman

Manfred began his strength athlete first with bodybuilding training, ultimately winning Austria's Strongest Man Contest seven times! Although bodybuilding style training was his first love, Manfred wanted to really test himself so he began training and competing as a strongman. Meeting South African Strongman legends Gerrit Badenhurst and Wayne Price, both massive men who made multiple World Strongest Man appearances. The very active strongman scene in South Africa was where Manfred cut his teeth. Manfred told Laurence he loved that the only opponent you really competed against in strongman is yourself.

After winning Austria's strongest man in 1989 and 1990, Manfred was invited to and competed at the 1991 World's Strongest Man contest where he debuted his most muscular physique. Manfred's peak years competing were 1993 and 1994, during which time he came in 2nd at the WSM Contest when he lost his focus and "stupidly looked over at Magnus ver Magnusson during the atlas stone load" and this cost him the title. He wistfully remarked at the lesson he learned the hard way: " Do your own thing and do it good. Don't worry about what others do."

During this time frame, Manfred competed in 40 competitions world wide, traveling with his fellow strongman to Highland games, exhibitions, as well as Strongman contests. Manfred described this period of time with a joy in his voice, stating that the strongman scene was full of strange characters who truly challenged each other in all the contested strength events. Each contest had unique events and equipment. The competitors were often surprised by what at least one or more event was.

In 1994 Manfred won Europe's Strongest Man, World Muscle Power Championships, Strongest Man on Earth Contest and the European Muscle Power Championships.

Manfred placed 8th in the 1991 WSM, 3rd in the 1993 WSM and 2nd at the 1994 WSM.

Manfred's Injuries

At the height of his career, Manfred severely injured his hips when he fell asleep at the wheel driving back from the world famous FIBO Fitness Exhibition. Luckily Manfred was driving a large, Mercedes Benz sedan when he hit a tree at a high rate of speed. Manfred had to be cut out of the luxury sedan but it probably saved his life. Manfred rehabilitated himself from this injury but then tore his bicep training his favorite event, the log press. Once this happened, Manfred retired because "he did not want to rehab or hurt himself anymore." He then focused his efforts on promoting the sport for a time.

In 2002, Manfred severely hurt himself as the result of a motorcycle crash, which left him in a wheel chair for two years and on crutches for ten more, with severe nerve damage. Being paralyzed for two years totally changed Manfred's mental outlook to one of gratitude.

In a YouTube clip on the Strength Universe Channel documents Manfred being interviewed following his comeback from the car accident at a Team Strongman contest in 1996, Manfred told the interviewer that he would have never survived the car crash if he had not been a competitive strongman, so he loves to give back to the sport and had to come back as a way to thank the fans.

Manfred's Arm Training Tips

Manfred built his world famous arms with short and intense workouts, lasting no more than 10 minutes. For biceps, Manfred favored dumbbell curls and for triceps, push downs on the lat machine. "Do the movements right." Manfred's book was entitled 10 Minutes to Massive Arms and sold well. At the 1994 Arnold Classic, Nick's Strength and Power YouTube channel reported that Manfred's arm was measured at 26" after he was able to pump his arms for 5 minutes. This measurement was over 3 times larger than his wrist, making him the first man to ever record such a message. Nick's claims Manfred's best bench press to be 628 lbs, his best squat to be 794lbs, and a best deadlift of 860lbs. Manfred was certified in 1997 on the famous Ironmind Company's #3 Captains of the Crush gripper, which is no easy feat.

Following being hit on his motorcycle by a car traveling at 80mph in 2002, Manfred has never lifted a weight again, per his doctors orders.

Greg Kovacs – The Canadian Colossus

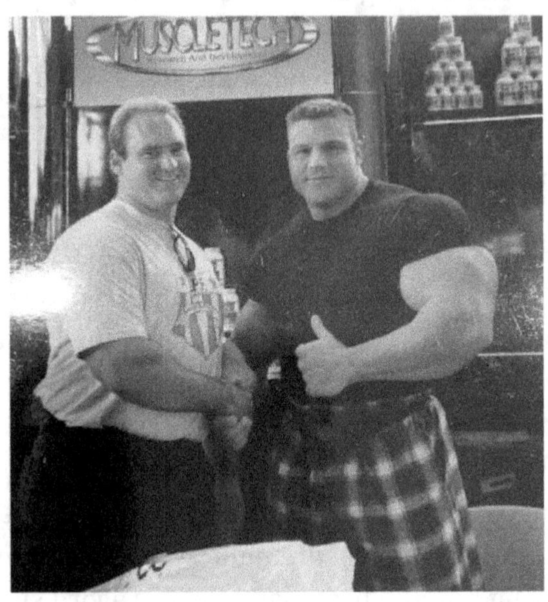

During the decade of the 1990s, before the dawn of the Internet, a new phenomenon entered the bodybuilding world, the 400lb off season bodybuilder! Although there were a few athletes associated with this mythical figure for body mass, the most famous was Canadian IFBB professional Greg Kovacs.

A YouTube video entitled Greg Kovacs- rare photos, that was posted by a channel Fitness by Matt, has pictures of Greg, provided by his sister Marta, beginning at age 13. Greg has obvious potential at that young age, with heavily muscled biceps. The second photo in this clip is of Greg in 1986, clearly showing great progress in his muscular development at age 18. A third photo from 1987 of Greg doing a most muscular pose shows incredible development as the author narrates that Greg was then at his full adult height of 6'2". A 1988 photo shows Greg, with help from a small framed spotter, bench pressing in a home gym with 585lbs of plates on the bar!

Fitness by Matt relates a tale told by Kovacs that he went to a powerlifting meet once and the best lift on the bench press was 430lbs. Greg was granted permission to attempt the weight and he did it for 19 repetitions! Continuing on with an analysis of the photos obtained from his family, there are photos of Greg as he went over 300 lbs for the first time and he has visible veins in his legs. A 1992 still shows Greg at 22 years old looking amazing in a Canadian provincial bodybuilding contest.

Nick's Strength and Power has done multiple YouTube videos on Greg, to include a 2017 piece entitled "the first bodybuilder to weigh 400 lbs., in the piece Nick claims that Greg got as high in bodyweight as 420lbs in the offseason. Nick says that Greg was 6'4" tall and competed at 330lbs on stage, with 26" arms in the offseason and 25" in contest condition, with a 70" chest and 35" quads when competing.

Despite not having competitive success, Greg was a financial success by receiving $10,000 dollar per appearances at his peak, of which he made many. That is when I met Greg, at the 1997 Mr. Olympia Contest Exposition in Long Beach, California. Nick posted another YouTube clip in which you see Greg have his arm measured at 25.5" while he is in good shape in the gym.

Greg Kovacs Video –The Strongest Bodybuilder Alive

Greg was the star of a bodybuilding video in which you can watch him workout at a Golds

Gym in Canada. The video was excellent quality and produced by Greg's main sponsor, Muscletech. In the 1990s the supplement industry was booming when anabolic steroids became controlled substances and all the major supplement companies had at least one bodybuilding star on their payroll to endorse their products. Muscletech was a major player in the industry by the late 1990s, buying up multiple page advertising spreads in all the bodybuilding magazines of the day.

The video opens with Greg incline pressing on a smith machine with 5 – 45 lb plates on each side. Greg does 3 repetitions on his own, then his spotter gives him just enough assistance for him to lock out additional repetitions in strict form. Greg then adds a 45 lb plate and does 5 repetitions with that huge amount of weight in strict form with what appears to be minimal assistance from his spotter. The incline bench Greg is pressing on appears to be set at 30 or 35 degrees.

The next exercise Greg does is a Hammer strength bench press machine it's 4 – 45 lb plates on each side of the machine. Greg smoothly and strictly presses this load for 9 reps and then finished the set with two partial repetitions, moving the weight from his chest and maintaining tension on his chest when he hit a sticking point and was unable to complete those last two repetitions. Greg continues the onslaught of his chest muscles with incline dumbbell flyes with 110lb dumbbells in each hand for high, strict repetitions on a bench set at approximately 25 degrees.

Day 2 begins with Greg training his massive biceps, with seated strict alternating dumbbell curls. It would appear Greg works up to over 70lb dumbbells. Like with his chest workout, Greg poses the body part he is training in between work sets. Next up, Greg does single arm preacher curls on an Icarian machine that is designed to use dual handles. Greg uses strict form and ten repetitions per set on this exercise. Tricep push downs are next, first with both arms on a straight bar, then he finished with single arm triceps extensions with an underhand grip.

Greg's wife described his diet on the video as breakfast being a large beef meal with 200 grams of carbohydrates such as oatmeal, bread or pancakes, along with 3 whole eggs. She summarized that Greg has 7 meals per day, alternating his protein sources throughout the day between beef, chicken and whole eggs. His carbohydrates are always potatoes, rice, yams and oatmeal.

The third day of training shown is Greg's leg workout and it begins with his easily doing the whole stack of a leg extension machine in a very strict manner. Next, Greg loads up an godly amount of 45 lb plates on a Nebula leg press and proceeds to do very strict and impressive repetitions with a huge amount of weight. A hack squat machine with 6 – 45 lb plates per side was the next exercise Greg expertly executed for high repetitions.

Greg described how he could press behind the neck 405 lbs for 6 to 8 repetitions when he was only 19. Seeing as my life's work has been powerlifting, I cannot say if Greg's claims of strength are true, but I will say that I met and spoke to Greg when I was totaling 1950 lbs in official powerlifting competitions and Greg was certainly one of the largest muscular humans I have ever met.

I have no reason to doubt that the weights he used in The Strongest Bodybuilder Alive were real. I do not know if Greg could have beaten Johnny Jackson, and I doubt he could have beaten Stan Efferding when he won the World's Strongest Pro Bodybuilder Title by officially totaling over 2300lbs raw in competition. Greg focused on bodybuilding training when he shot that video so it would not be fair to compare the two athletes.

Greg's training philosophy is to go as heavy as he can for full range of motion repetitions for 6 to 8 reps. Greg said he trains each body part only once per week. Greg said he had to learn to train instinctively, knowing when to work the muscle next.

Greg's 4th training day is shoulders and he begins his session with the Hammer Strength press behind the neck machine, doing 7 reps with 5- 45lb plates and 1- 25 lb plate on each side. Greg's form is textbook as always. Seated strict side dumbbell laterals with 70lb bells were next, with Greg's form impeccable and strict as hell. Icarian side deltoid raises followed, with Greg pushing the exercise to failure.

Day 5 is a back day, beginning with Icarian rear deltoid flyes with the whole stack, strict for high repetitions. Strict dumbbell shrugs with straps for high reps are up next on the menu for Mr. Kovacs. Underhand grip pull downs with the whole weight stack and an added 45 lb plate were attacked next, with strict form and a great range of motion. Greg's last exercise was one arm Hammer strength seated rows with 5- 45 lb plates on each side for, many full, strict repetitions.

Greg passed away in 2013 at the age of 44 from heart failure, two weeks after he had a heart surgery. I am glad that I got to meet him and congratulate him on his success in person in 1997. I hope he left this earth knowing that he influenced countless iron addicts with his size, personality and well thought out training. May he Rest In Peace.

Richard Schoenberger – Big Daddy from Southern Cali

I have been fortunate in my life time to meet and experience many amazing human beings, specifically many who are interested in training for strength improvement. When I relocated to Southern California in 1991, I first lived in Whittier, which had a number of really cool hardcore gyms within a short drive of each other. Knowing my Powerlifting history as I do, I knew that Pat Casey, the first man to officially bench 600lbs and total 2000, at one time owned a gym in Norwalk, which is adjacent to Whittier. Pat's gym was long gone, but I soon discovered that the American Eagle Gym was located in Norwalk and it had something no other gym in the World had in 1993- two raw 600lb Bench pressers.

As of this article, anyone who is interested in hard training and has an internet connection knows who CT Fletcher is- but not everyone knows of **CT's training partner**, Richard Schoenberger. There are two awesome videos on <u>CT Fletcher's YouTube channel </u>in which he introduces Richard to the world and explains to all how Richard is more than a training partner to him, he is a brother. The first video details how CT calls Richard the Silverback and how they trained together on Monday nights at the American Eagle Gym in Norwalk, which at that time was owned by the super supportive Sherry Houston. Monday night was bench night and I was fortunate to observe their workouts for over a year while they were nearing their peak in strength in 1993.

Richard humbly speaks on this first YouTube clip and he describes how he is a husband, father, and son before he is a lifter. He began weight training for football as a high school sophomore weighing only 165 lbs – he would increase his bodyweight by almost 200 at the peak of his bench pressing career.

Rich, long a professional engineer by trade, recalled that he **gained 30 lbs of bodyweight per year once he began training.** Richard provided CT with some interesting information such as how he pushed a Camaro two miles and after High School he lifted a Volkswagen to win a bet with his dad. CT stated that he could bench press 405lbs when he turned 18, which Richard added that he benched 425 lbs when he was 16 years young!

Richard humbly said that he was very fortunate to be born strong as his father was unbelievably strong from working on automobiles his entire life without mechanical lifts. Richard was also heavily influenced by his High School Football Coach Hennigan who started him lifting weights.

Richard was as good a student as a he was a lifter, graduating High School with straight As in every subject. Richard played Junior College Football at Cerritos Junior College then earned a scholarship to play football at California Polytechnic College in San Luis Obispo, California. Upon graduation, Rich began his professional career at Rockwell, a huge aerospace company located in Southern California. As fate would have it, Rockwell had a great fitness center that was run by former Powerlifting World Record holder Dave Shaw. Dave organized a company bench press contest which Richard won, beginning his streak of 14 years of being undefeated in bench press contests.

Richard's best official bench press was 625lbs raw, which was a world record in the American Amateur Athletic Union. Richard never wore a bench press shirt, at time when they were the most popular. There is an awesome YouTube video which is one of the old Ned Low's Powerlifter Video Magazine editions which shows Richard benching at the American Eagle and benching 615lbs. Richard and I lifted at the 1995 California State Powerlifting Championships where I beat Mike O'hearn and he benched over 600 raw as CT cheers him on. These video clips are on my YouTube channel, Paul L.

Richard humbly thanks his family and training partners for their years of loyal support which let him succeed. He also thanked CT on video for their Monday night battles that made each of them greater. After meeting at a Halloween Powerlifting contest at the American Eagle, these two "polar opposites became the best of friends." CT intensely described how when he went into the hospital for his heart transplant, Richard was there along with his wife Leslie, because as CT says:

"They are closer than blood."

The number one thing you will take away from learning about Richard is the fulfillment you will feel as a person due to the bonds you form with your training partners, not the records, the magazine appearances, or the places you experienced when you traveled to compete.

My favorite Richard story has nothing to do with lifting weights at all. In the summer of 1993, my buddy Eric Deroian and I went to the Cowboy Boogie, which was a nightclub in Anaheim off I -5 that must have been over 100,000 square feet and packed when we arrived. As we made our way through the sea of humanity that was the crowd, all of sudden the people had surrounded someone who was dancing their ass off to "Whoop there it is". You guessed it, Richard at all of 350 lbs, as wide as he was tall, had the impromptu Soul Train spotlight on him as he moved like Prince to an adoring and appreciative crowd.

Art Labare – A Powerlifting Legend You Need to Know

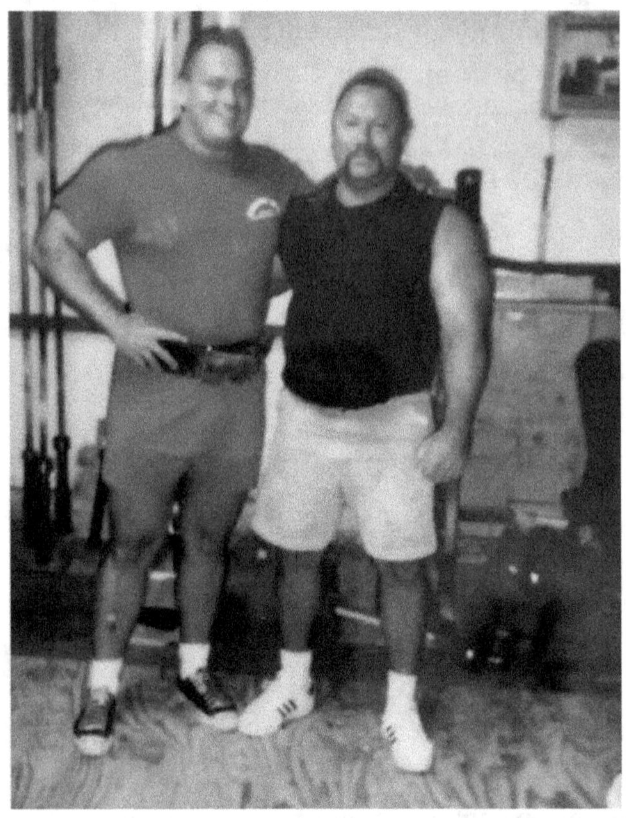

In life you will meet many people, some you like, a few you love, those you hate- especially as you get older, and the rest are all just passing through, pedestrian in their importance to your life. Us strength athletes are unique in that we have other individuals in our lives who leave an indelible mark- training partners. I have had many training partners over my 36 years of serious weight training, many whom I love, all I like, and one that has passed away. Of all these training partners, Art Labare stands out above all others for his character, dedication, and performance on the platform and in the gym. Art is 8 years older than I am, so some of the things he went through as we trained together did not register with me until later when I had kids of my own and more time constraints.

Art's best lifts are 876 628 793, all done at National or World Class Meets in the late 90s through 2004. It is pretty fitting that Art hit his best total in 2004 after I relocated to Dallas and our other partner had serious personal demons which led to his untimely demise that same year. Art did not need anyone to do his best lifting.

I first met Art in 1995 at the USPF California State Meet which Art entered but did not lift anywhere near his capability. Art was training at that time with Brian Meek, Rick Purchase, and Gary Garcia in South Orange County, usually at either PowerHouse Gym Fountain Valley or World Gym in Tustin. I trained at Uptown Gym in Whittier with Gary Hogan, Mike Morgan, Al Morentin, Ray Cosio, and Ron Perkins. Art whopped mine and most everyone else's ass at the WPC Can Ams in Vegas in 1996, but I still was not training with him. In late 1997, I had lost some training partners, but the final straw was when Gary told me that he could not keep up with my schedule and that he needed a break from our usual Monday, Tuesday, Thursday night 7 to 9 pm sessions as well as from our Saturday lower body assault from 9 to noon. I was out of sorts until I saw Art and we decided we would begin training in my garage with his crew. Art had torn his biceps at the 1997 APF Seniors and I had the shittiest meet of my PL career in the fall of 97. Something had to change for both of us.

By forming an alliance with Art, I had the most productive Powerlifting years of my life from 1998 to 2003. My platform performances were well earned and important to me- despite the fact that many of them are not reflected in the website OpenPowerlifting-yet. But this article is about Art and what a true training partner can mean to another lifter.

On January 1, 1998, Art and I began our assault with him showing me his 5, 10, 15, broke workout which was taking a weight on the bench and repping it for five, ten, fifteen and then to failure for reps. I used 315 and Art did as well. I sucked after the set with 15 reps but Art hit approximately 25 good reps with three plates. Like 90%

of our training, this was done raw. As an aside, Art was phenomenal at reps in the bench. One summer Saturday, Art repped 225 lbs for 46 full reps at the grand opening of a South Bay Harley Davidson Shop as part of their grand opening, barbecue type bench contest. Coupled with the hot body contest and So Cal scenic crowd, that was a great day.

This impromptu bench contest was not the most memorable one I ever saw Art compete in however. None to compare to a bench meet that was held as part of a grand opening of a new 24 hour fitness in Orange County. As per the norm, we were close to finishing up a max effort lower body workout in my garage in Yorba Linda when a call came in as to why Art was not at the bench meet set to begin at 1 pm. We had not known about the contest until the call, but all Art had to hear was that Cocco, a decent bencher who thought very highly of himself was entered and had assumed, rather publicly, that Art had ducked his challenge in his own backyard of OC. We proceeded to pile in to Art's truck and within a few hours Art had benched over 500 and set the record straight.

There was a time I sold a 2 hour video tape of our workouts at Yorba Barbell online. After he reviewed the tape in his monthly PLUSA column, Dr Ken Leistner sold a bunch of tapes for me that allowed me to buy more equipment. The most famous moment in the tape is when the crew is doing floor presses off of my not bolted down power rack. Art is top dog of the day and is floor pressing over 500lbs, when the bar gets stuck under the j-cup on the way to lockout and the rack is lifted off the floor and locked out with the bar. Anyone who has seen this tape has remarked about how amazing Art's lifting is.

Whenever Art was challenged he was surely at his best, much like a wounded animal, Art would get these dark, shark like eyes, and he would unleash everything he had. Art was on a short hiatus due to his bicep tear when he rode up to a full garage one evening. A newer lifter who did not know any better asked Art, what are you doing here with your bicep hurt? Art took one disgusted look at the guy, shoved him to the side and proceeded to grab the power

rack chin up bar to bang out 12 perfect chins. Then Art got into the mouth's face and exclaimed that no one should doubt his arm.

99% of the time, Art was cool, calm, and quiet as many of his Yorba mates, myself included were far more verbose. Art's display of raw emotion would also boil over if he felt a friend was being questioned. In 2000, Art handled me when I won the heavy weight best lifter at the Santa Barbara East Beach Open, but lost the overall to 148er Scott Layman. Scott let us know he was pound for pound the man-and Art leaned in towards him and hissed – "Remember, when people go to the circus they go to see the lions Scott, not the ants."

At the 1998 APF Cal States in Fresno, Art dominated the meet and when he received his award, he hit a mocking most muscular because 2nd place finisher Joe DeAngelis (RIP) had been Mr America and decided to hit poses after each of his lifts. Art had been mentored by **Roger Estep, Terry McCormick and Dave Shaw**– Powerlifting royalty who taught Art and all of us at Yorba to respect the sport and your time on the platform.

Art had a quiet, non-conformist streak in him. Maybe it was because he grew up a stones throw from the famous Zuvers Gym in Costa Mesa. It could have been because after graduating from high school Art moved to Hawaii for a year to become a professional surfer. Art would sew his own bench shirts together and if he did have to buy one, he would spray paint over the Inzer logo because they did not sponsor him yet they sponsored teammates such as Josh and myself. Art is a very successful drywall contractor who worked his ass off to

build a company which afforded he and his family a comfortable lifestyle. Art's generosity went far beyond his family, as his company sponsored my trip to handle him at the inaugural WPO show in Daytona Beach. If you look closely, you can see me putting on Art's straps at that meet in the new Westside vs the World documentary.

Art was always there for me, at every meet, regardless of whether he was competing or not. I strayed from the way so to speak and started doing competitive Strongman training in 2001 following a knee injury. Art was supportive of me, even though his strength goals were strictly Powerlifting. Once I came back to Powerlifting, Art had my back, flying up to Sacramento to be there for my first official 800lb squat. Same thing for my first official 2000lb total, Art was there at Universal Studios but not competing.

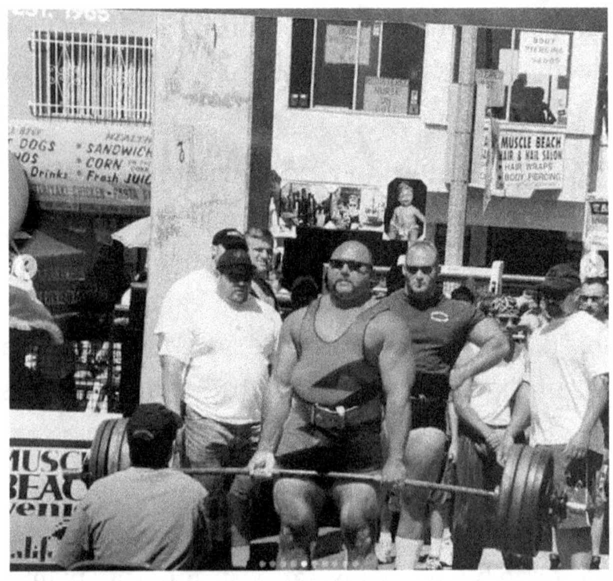

THE PICTURE AT VENICE SHOW ART PULLING IN A SINGLET HE FOUND WHICH I NAMED THE

SCREAMING TOMATO."

"The picture at Venice show Art pulling in a singlet he found which I named the screaming tomato." – Paul

The one thing I recall most about Art's demeanor was his quiet confidence. Art knew what he wanted to do, made up in his mind his goals and achieved them. When training together, I followed more of a Westside Conjugate style with box squats and various

Max Effort exercises. Art free squatted his sets and did not do the zercher squats, kneeling squats and pull throughs I enjoyed.

We all did variations of speed pulls for our deadlifts at my garage- all conventional and with lower percentages for singles. I had 7 men who trained in my gym who officially pulled over 744, but the biggest pull ever done in the gym was 700 and that did not give us the training effect we wanted.

Louie Simmons

I first read about Louie Simmons in 1987 in Powerlifting USA Magazine. Louie wrote a series of articles in the late 1980s which I read but did not really understand. I did not apply any of the concepts that Louie discussed and I trained in the traditional progressive overload method that was popular at that time.

I did learn that Louie had been powerlifting since the early 1970s and was a pioneer of the sport. He ultimately totaled the elite total requirement for 5 different weight classes- something I believe only the immortal Fred Hatfield had done during his illustrious career. Louie was a National level competitor in the early 1970s and would go on to set open division top ten records in squat (920) bench (600) deadlift (715) and total into his 50s and 60s! But I am getting ahead of myself.

In approximately 1993, Louie began writing articles that were published again after a 3 year hiatus of his sharing knowledge with the only Powerlifting Magazine in the world at that time.

The articles also contained an advertisement for Louie's video tape series with a tape for each lift entitled squat secrets,bench press secrets and deadlift secrets. I received these video tapes for Christmas 1993 and they were instrumental in me learning about the Westside Barbell method.

I had relocated to Southern California and at first I was disillusioned with the training atmosphere I found there. I lived in various parts of So Cal, but never found a gym or a training crew that inspired or interested me. I received Louie's tapes in 1993 and I studied everything I could about him and his Westside Barbell System. Louie has said many times that when he started powerlifting he only had a power rack and an AM radio as his training partners. I was the same, except I had Louie's tapes and articles.

With Louie's information, I began applying everything he taught whoever was wise enough to listen. I had gotten to the stage where I could squat 600 bench 385 and deadlift 650, before I began Westside training. I had stagnated for a few years and knew, as Louie says, everything works, but nothing works forever. I trained Westside style on my own and hit my first 1700lb total in late 1994. Soon, I met a crew of powerlifters and relocated to be near the gym they trained at in Whittier, California.

I convinced really good local lifters to train with me and we followed the Westside system as best we could not actually training there. Everyone who trained with us at Yorba Barbell got stronger. I placed at that Men's Senior Nationals and Louie Simmons became familiar with my name. I gave back to the sport by writing articles about my training partners Art LaBare and Josh Bryant. I competed at the meets that Westside went to, but I never met Louie.

The first time I met Louie was in 1999 at the IPA Seniors at York Pennsylvania. None of my training partners could travel with me from California to Pennsylvania so I had to find a crew to warm up with for my lifts and to get my gear on. I had sent Louie Simmons a copy of a Jon Coles 2370 total on VHS that year as a way to thank him for helping me total elite in 1998. I had been trading emails with Westsider Bob Youngs who was at the meet in York along with Matt Smith, Jimmie Ritchie, John Stafford, Todd Brock and Louie Simmons himself!

I introduced myself to Louie and he said he knew me from my articles in PLUSA as well as from the Cole tape I had mailed him. Louie invited me to warm up with Westside- which I was honored to do. Once Louie said I was in, I was in the Westside inner circle that day. I had a good day- not my best, but I placed 5th in the 308s and I did out total Matt Smith who would go on to win a WPO belt in a few years. Bob Youngs has since died of cancer and I never got to lift with any of those same Westside lifters, but Louie took me in when I needed help and he validated everything I had ever heard about his high character.

I continued to follow everything that Louie and Westside released as far as information, even when I competed in Strongman in 2001 and 2002. The next time I spoke to Louie Simmons was in 2007 when my training partner Mike Martin hurt his shoulder and needed some advice. I called Louie and left a message about the situation as well as Mike's phone number. Later that day, Louie called Mike and talked with him for over an hour about how he should fix his shoulder. Mike has benched over 400 raw for over 30 years and attributes Louie's advice and training system as the reason for his success and longevity.

I have not spoken to Louie in over 14 years now, but if I needed him he would be there for me. Today his website and podcasts are still loaded with information I learn from. Louie invited me to train at Westside more than once, but I have not done so yet.

Remember, Louie has said many times he regretted never going to the Original Westside in Culver City during the early 1970s- he only dreamt of going because work and life responsibilities kept him in Ohio. He built his dream gym and system there- I suggest you do the same. Louie often said he was envious of powerlifting legend Roger Estep who left Ohio with a 1600lb total at 198 and became the world record holder in the total by training with original Westside legend George Frenn. Imagine how lucky I was to move to California and befriend Roger before he passed away.

Louie Simmons is everything that is right about powerlifting. He has dedicated his life to the sport. He has given so much of himself to anyone interested in furthering the sport or their own lifts. He undeniably built the premiere powerlifting club in the World for almost two decades. Personally, Louie gave my life direction when I was a young, impressionable lifter with no answers to my training problems and plateaus. After I followed Louie's advice, my strength dreams came true. The only thing I wonder about when it comes to Louie Simmons is, who will replace him as the premiere strength coach in powerlifting once he is no longer here?

Joe Ladnier – Mass Monster with a 24" Neck

Joe "The Lad"Joe Ladnier burst onto the Powerlifting scene in 1983, when 19 years old, he won the U.S. Senior National Men's Powerlifting Championships at 242 lbs with a squat of 832 a bench of 556 and a deadlift of 788. He beat such legends as Fred Hatfield and Jim Cash. In doing so, Joe set open men's world records and teenage world records that have stood for over 30 years. Joe was interviewed by Starting Strength's Mark Rippetoe in 2014, and the three part interview appears on YouTube. Joe is extremely articulate and has a great recollection of his powerlifting career as well as so many fantastic lifters he trained with, knew or competed against.

Joe won the teenage nationals three times. Joe, Aka the Mississippi Monster, worked for

Larry Pacifico, managing one of his Dayton, Ohio gyms, his mail order business and was in Pacifico's ads which appeared in Powerlifting USA Magazine. Larry taught Joe how to correctly add assistance exercises to his training, specifically bodybuilding exercises to complement his powerlifting training.

Joe relocated to Florida after living in Georgia for a short time. While in Florida he was part of the famous Suncoast Gym Team which had such members as Rick Weil and Bob Chrosniak. While training there, **Joe benched a 600lb raw bench** at the Florida State Championships. Two days after this bench performance, Joe detached his patella tendon and tore his ACL and MCL. This injury altered the course of Joe's lifting career for years. The injury occurred in 1986, after Joe switched from his normal wide stance to a closer stance at the coaching of Fred Hatfield.

Joe felt that the switch to close stance would result in a world record as he squatted 600lbs for 20 reps with knee wraps and a belt. A few workouts later Joe was squatting 900lbs when he tore his patella.

While in Florida, Joe became a police officer with a Sheriff's Department. He did not talk about how or why his law enforcement career did not last longer than 5 years.

In 1988, Joe entered and won the U.S. Drug Free Nationals and the Drug Free World Championships as well.

One of the most successful transitions to Masters and raw competition later in his life. Joe recalled that he took the entire 90s off from competition to focus on his family. He said he always trained during that time period but he did not compete due to his family commitments.

Joe said that he was able to lift at the same World meet as his teenage daughter! After winning her class, his daughter told him that she was not interested in lifting again. Joe said that his son defeated future IPF Champion Ian Bell at a teenage meet, but that as of 2014, his son had recently started training again and was 21 at that time.

As recently as a few years ago Joe benched 525 raw and deadlifted 700 raw as well. There are numerous clips on YouTube that show Joe's masters level power as well as his younger, senior nationals performances. Joe said he had focused on the bench with a shirt when he came back to powerlifting in the early 2000s and hit an 825 officially!

Joe was on the cover of numerous Powerlifting magazines during his career, specifically Powerlifting USA and Monster Muscle.

Joe recalled impressive lifters he trained with and he described how he trained with Jim Cash and saw Jim deadlift 10 strict repetitions with 700lbs! One year at the Hawaii Invitational, Lee Moran missed a 600 lb raw bench, after squatting well over 900lbs. The next day, they went to the gym and Lee benched the 600lbs raw. Lee was Joe's height of 5'7" but outweighed Joe by 90lbs at 330lbs!

A 1984 Powerlifting USA article by fantastic author Ron Fernando described Joe's 18 month meteoric rise in strength, up until he became 20 years of age. Ron detailed how Joe entered his first meet at 160lbs in 1979 and did 350 290 430 lbs. The most interesting fact of this performance was the Joe had never performed a squat or a deadlift prior to the contest! Joe had bench pressed before the contest but his strength primarily came from gymnastics training- much like his 80s rival and later mentor, Fred Hatfield. Joe's first mentor was a man named Larry Plumlee who was great lifter in Mississippi where Joe grew up. He guided Joe from a 1350 total at 165 to an 1802lb total at 198 in 2 years!

In 1984 when Joe was winning National Championships and competing at the worlds, he would squat on Sundays and Wednesdays. Joe loved Soviet style jump training to supplement his squat workouts. Fernando detailed a workout at the time that he worked up to 865 for 3 reps in a squat suit, knee wraps and a belt, followed up by sets of 3 second pause squats for triples up to 715lbs! Joe would perform walkouts with between 900 and 950 lbs. Joe would at times take the walkout weight and do a half squat to feel the weight.

On Joe's light squat night he would go up to 405 for 1, using perfect form and explosiveness. Both leg workouts included 3 sets of 10 reps of box jumps, leg extensions and leg curls. Joe boasted a best vertical box jump of 48"! Joe was able to maintain his gymnast flexibility and was able to complete full splits even as a 900lb squatter! This is very similar to Ronnie Coleman.

Joe's bench press training was similar to his squat work, as he had one heavy bench press workout per week- with the heavy session on Sunday working up an inverted pyramid to a set with 518 for 3, followed by long 3 second pause work with the bar high on the chest with up to 407 for 3 reps. His muscle memory workout was Thursday, during which he would work up to 315 for a rep or 3with perfect and explosive form. On both days, his assistance would be cambered incline benches for 5 to 8 reps with up to 250lbs , and flyes with 70lb dumbbells.

The day after his bench workouts, Joe loved to do arm workout superset style with up to 305 for 6 reps on the Ez curl bar to his chin with tricep extensions! Joe has amazing arms- I have seen them, and he built them with ez bar curls, push downs, dumbbell curls and the extensions.

Joe has had the hardest time with the deadlift, which he trains on Wednesday with the same type of inverted pyramid he uses on his other lifts. Ron described a workout that peaked with a top triple of 730 for 3 reps! Joe had success with block deadlifts with the weight positioned below his knees, with a huge PR of 825 for 3. Shrugs and hyperextensions with a hundred pound plate for 3 sets of 10 reps.

Joe described to Ron that as he got stronger, he got more and more in control of his emotions. The Lad was able to stay in a state of Zen calm that was as impressive as his rapid strength gains.

I only met Joe once, at the 2003 APF Senior National Championships at Universal Studios Hollywood. Joe did not lift that day, even though he was the defending National champion from 2002. Joe was extremely impressive in person, with more muscles on his 5'7" frame than I had seen on almost any person.

A review of OpenPowerlifting.Org documents that Joe went on to win one GPC World championship as well as numerous SPF National Championships between 2009 and 2016.

Joe's Instagram account, thejoeladnier, shows a healthy and happy looking Joe today. On August 7, 2021, Joe exhibited his Alabama Hall of Fame Plaque on his page. What a great honor to a very worthy recipient. Joe's Instagram shows a happy family man who is far more jacked than almost any 60 year old I have ever seen. I suggest you follow the Lad's training philosophy if you seek to train and compete successfully for over 4 decades.

Brooks Kubik

2021 marks the 25th year of the release of Dinosaur Training by Brooks Kubik. Although Mr. Kubik has gone through publicized changes in his training style during this quarter of a century, this article is going to focus on his 1996 book which has had such a profound influence on strength training.

The book is an examination of the correct philosophy that needs to be applied by anyone that seeks to improve their physical strength. Brooks, a lawyer by trade- i.e a paid arguer, certainly knows how to examine an issue from every possible angle. The result of Mr. Kubik's analysis is a thorough description of all the possible training methods and programs that can applied to forge a body with strength, power, and muscular development.

Dr. Ken Leistner had written about, demonstrated on video and championed hard, intense training in his writings published in Ironman, Powerlifting USA, Muscular Development, Milo, and his own Newsletter The Steel tip- beginning in the early 1970s through the 2000s.

Leistner influenced a generation of trainees to include Kubik, and received mention in Dinosaur training, specifically in a fantastic chapter entitled "Death sets!"

The training landscape in 1996, as evidenced by the contemporary Bodybuilding magazines escalating arms race with total pages published along with ESPN,which had numerous bodybuilding training shows in the am were not promoting intense training, odd object lifting, power rack work, grip strength, partials, heavy singles, or thick bar implementation.

Dinosaur training is a self described throat punch to the weak, mainstream training philosophies that were being promoted in the glossy magazines and training shows filmed on the beach.

Just as Dinosaur training rolled off the printing press, ESPN 2 was launched and the broadcasts of the Worlds Strongest Man began, introducing the viewers to log lifting, barrel lifting, sand bag pressing, stone lifting and thick bar implements such as Ironmind's Appollons Axle.

Milo was promoting dinosaur style training, so a revolution in training began. Today, shows that document how MMA fighters and star football players train have their roots in Dinosaur training. The palatial weight facilities of today, with chains, tires, sleds, odd objects, thick implements, farmer's walk equipment, and sand bags all were popularized and promoted by Dinosaur Training.

Dinosaur training has programs that are applicable to every level of trainee. When I was totally focused on competitive powerlifting, the chapters on mental training helped me the most, allowing me to total elite in 1998 and finish in the top 5 in the United States in contests between 1996 and 2006. I attribute my competitive successes in the decade following first reading Dinosaur Training to the philosophy of embracing training as hard as physically possible.

Later in my lifting journey, after I had suffered serious injuries requiring surgeries, I was able to come back and set State Records thanks to the rack work programs derailed by Brooks. Allowing me to train without minimal eccentric stress allowed my numerous tendon reattachments to heal and be as strong as prior to my injuries. Rack work coupled with thick bar work, dissipated stress over my joints which took a beating for 20 years to reach the top. I can do higher volume pressing with an axle as well as develop a stronger grip with thick bar curls. The current trend in strict curls was written about extensively by Kubik 25 years ago!

The chapters in Dinosaur training are short, focused and as subtle as a sledgehammer. The book culminates with multiple chapters stressing the mental aspect of correct weight training, with a focus on extreme concentration.

One of my favorite chapters is entitled:

"Do it for yourself."

In this day of lifting for Internet likes and Instagram posts, this chapter certainly is a common sense approach that is beautifully brutal in it's simplicity.

I cannot stress enough how much knowledge, inspiration, and physical culture history a serious trainee can learn from owning this book and referring to it frequently. As I mentioned at the beginning of this article, Mr. Kubik sells numerous training books and programs, but you could have a lifetime of guidance in how to correctly change just by following the information in Dinosaur Training alone.

Oldtime-Strength Stars you have to know

Doug Hepburn: King of the Curl!

During 2020, the strict curl went viral with Larry Wheels and former NFL legend James Harrison releasing videos of their respective impressive strict curls. Over 70 years ago, one of the strongest men of his time, Doug Hepburn was able to curl 255lbs/115kg! This curl was done in 1959. For contextual purposes, Doug Hepburn was the 1953 World Weightlifting Super Heavyweight Champion, with a then highest total ever of 1030 lb total. I think that gives the reader a good understanding of the strength of Hepburn. Doug's all time best strength performances all occurred while he was 285lbs and had an arm measurement of

21.5."

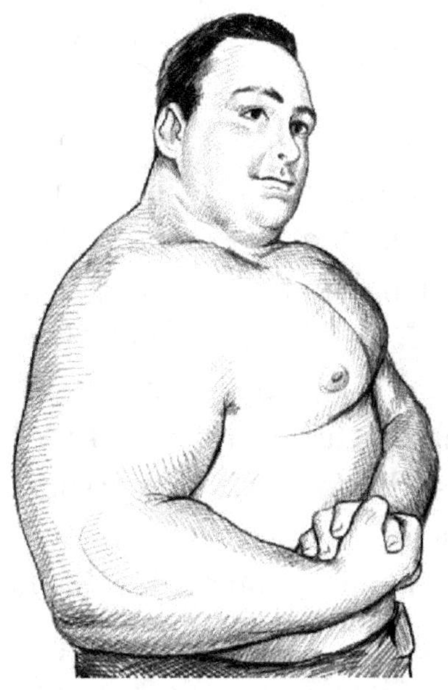

An Ironman article **'Developing Curling Power'** written by Doug in March, 1961 explained his training philosophy in building such amazing curling strength. This fascinating article begins with an

extremely detailed description of how to grip the bar, specifically the best grip width and wrist position to take to begin a correctly performed set of curls.

Hepburn described curl grip width as different for each individual, with the hands being just outside contact with the thighs when the bar is help. Doug said that a false grip should never be used when curling and that the bar should be gripped as close to the wrist as possible-this will give the lifter the best leverage possible.

Doug's words from his 1961 piece, tell the lifter to perform each rep with as much explosive power as possible. The faster you begin a repetition from the starting position, the greater the chance you will power through the sticking point. Also when you curl explosively there is less chance that your form will deteriorate to a lean back position. Keeping the elbows in as close as possible to the sides was stressed by Hepburn, as well as not exhaling the breath you took prior to picking up the bar until you were past the sticking point.

As for sets and repetitions, Doug found that a series of low repetition sets combined with a limited amount of heavy singles will result in the greatest lifting strength. To warm up for his series of repetition sets, Doug would begin with a set of 5 reps then increase the weight so that a single can be comfortably curled. Hepburn told Ironman that he was rest for 3 to 5 minutes between repetition sets and singles. Doug would add weight and do a single, then add more weight and do three singles. His goal was to build up to 5 singles with the weight he curled for 3 singles. Hepburn heavily stressed progress and said that the lifter should continue with the 3 singles- progressing to 5 singles indefinitely. The aforementioned warm up curls should be adjusted proportionately as a lifters singles increase.

Hepburn described a variation of his curl program in which he would focus on 3 sets of 3 reps- building these sets up to 5 sets of 5 repetitions. Both Doug's programs were as simple and brutal as a throat punch.

How many lifters today do you see strict curling 255 lbs?

Have pressed a pair of 170 lb. dumbbells simultaneously in training here and pressed two 160's at a show in Oakland, California in 1952. While there I pressed a man well in excess of 300 lbs. to arms' length overhead.

CURL

On May 20, 1959, I curled 255 in good form and also swing-curled 300; this was done at a show here in Vancouver in the presence of AAU officials. Bodyweight 285 pounds.

I have held a pair of 100 pound dumbbells out from the sides, at shoulder level. This was done here in Vancouver in 1952.

Have also held a 150 lb. barbell out in front of the shoulders for three seconds. Have also held out to the side two plates, 45 lbs. each; a belt was passed through the plates and I held the plates by the little finger of my right hand passed through the belt.

I have dropped a 325 lb. bar from overhead and caught it in the crooks of the elbows; this, I might add, is rather painful and not recommended to those with tender skin.

SQUAT

I was handicapped in this lift because of my bad leg and when I first started training I was convinced that I would never squat with heavy poundages. However, my thighs were not affected to any great extent so I managed to squat with some respectable weights. My record squat is 760; this was done in training here in Vancouver, 1957. I also did a full squat and remained in the low position for five seconds before arising. Have also squatted with 600 for ten consecutive repetitions.

Have dead-lifted 740 with the use of steel hooks attached to my hands. I have always had difficulty holding onto heavy weights with my hands, hence the clips. However, I have never specialized on the dead-lift and I feel that I could do more in the accepted style.

BENCH PRESS

My best bench press is 580; this was done with an extreme wide grip and a slight bounce at the chest. My best public performance was 550 lbs. at Portland in 1957. This lift was done easily and I made the mistake of jumping to 600 lbs. I almost had the bar at arms' length and I lost control of it and it came down on my NECK. There were no spotters. I held the weight off my neck with my arms until the bar could be removed. I severely tore the shoulders doing this; however, I consider myself lucky. It must have affected my vocal chords as all I could do was whisper for a few weeks. (I guess a lot of married fellows would wish something like this on their wives, on a permanent basis.)

I have bench pressed 525 and have stopped the bar on the chest for three seconds. I also used a closer grip for this lift.

Have done 500 lbs. for 7 consecutive repetitions in training. I think I did 5 or 6 repetitions at a Montreal show for Ben Weider in 1955.

My present measurements are: chest 59, normal arm 21½, waist 46, forearm 16 (not goose-neck), thighs 32, neck 20, wrists 8½. Bodyweight 280 lbs. Have enclosed a photo taken just recently, this is all I have at present.

Yours sincerely,
Doug Hepburn

A few of us took pleasure in recording and analyzing the feats of old time strong men and never in our wildest dreams did we conjure anything like Doug Hepburn or the super-heavyweight lifters that followed him, right up to the present. Hepburn had no science, no fast lightning style to drop himself under a weight and, in addition, he had a physical handicap. The specialized feats of old time strong men, which were little altars at which we worshipped, were all surpassed by Hepburn. He did not specialize on these feats; he was just a man of immense all around muscular power, with good muscular reflexes, and a dedication to strength. He proved, without really trying to, that he could display greater strength feats than Swoboda, Moerke, Steinborn, Assirati, Maier, Grafl, Goerner, Saxon, Inch, and as Joe Weider once wrote: "One of these days, the full story of Hepburn will be told and when it is it will serve forever as an inspiration to us all — for it will tell how a boy overcame a physical handicap to become the GREATEST OF THEM ALL."

Many people are unwilling to concede that Hepburn was the equal of John Davis in the Olympic lifts. In a way this was true because Doug was handicapped in the clean,

On that day in May 1959 he did his monster strict curl, Hepburn also did a swing curl with 300lbs/136kg!

Simple works and is beautifully brutal. Hepburn's curls are documented as the heaviest on record done with a straight bar, as many heavy curls were done with EZ curl bars.

A history of the curl

I had the pleasure of training with CT Fletcher at the American Eagle Gym in Norwalk, California in 1993 at the time he held the recognized world strict curl record of 232lbs. CT's arms were in the same class as Ted Arcidi, Ryan Kennelly, and Greg Kovacs as the biggest arms I have ever seen.

Bill Kazmaier, Arnold Schwarzenegger, Larry Wheels, and CT Fletcher are known for their ponderous curl poundages, with Russian Denis Cyplenkov receiving credit for the all time heaviest strict curl with 249lbs, as seen on more than a few YouTube channels because everyone loves the curl. Although it is rumored that Kazmaier curled 440lbs, there is no documented proof of this alleged feat, as opposed to most of Katz's strength records which occurred at the WSM or National Powerlifting Championships and are beyond question.

The owner of neckberg.com reported that he recently watched a YouTube video in which

Golden Era Strength historian Ric Drasin interviewed Chuck Mahoney who claims he saw Strength legend Chuck Aherns do three concentration curls with 185lbs. There is no documented proof of this claim but it is interesting none the less.

Arnold Schwarzenegger curled heavily to build the best looking biceps in history, with noted German strength historian telling this website's owner that in 1966 Arnold did a Powerlifting contest at which he squatted 150 kilos, benched 140 kilos, and curled 100 kilos.

Hepburn is credited by Wikipedia with a 260lb curl, while he did a 255lb curl at a competition that was administered by the AAU in 1959. According to the website <u>American Powerlift Evolution. Net,</u> the first AAU sanctioned curl contest was in 1954. Within 5 years of it's origin, the Canadian Colossus of Curls was the World Record holder!

High Praise from Joe Weider

Magazine mogul Joe Weider said this to describe Doug Hepburn: "A few of us took pleasure in recording and analyzing the feats of the old time strongmen and never in our wildest dreams did we conjure up anything like Doug Hepburn. Hepburn had no science, no lighting fast descent to drop under a weight and in addition he had a physical handicap. The specialized feats of old time strongmen, which were altars at which we worshipped, were all surpassed by Hepburn. He did not specialize on these feats; he was just a man of immense all around muscular power, with good muscular reflexes, and a dedication to strength." Weider continued: " He needs no experience, no years of specialized training, he can just do them."

Mac Batchelor – THE UNDEFEATED ARM WRESTLER

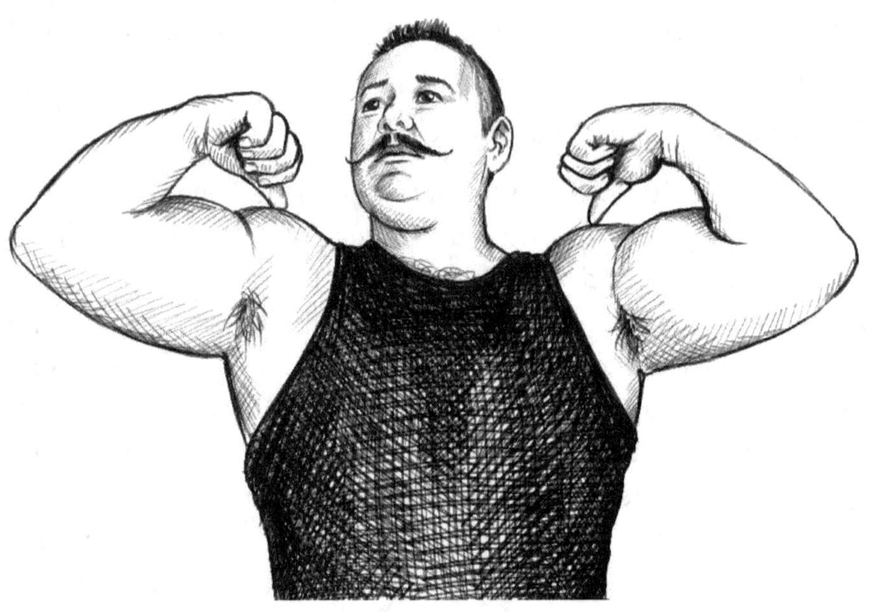

Ian Gordon Bachelor was known as Mac. Mighty Mac was undefeated in arm wrestling from 1931 to 1956. Muscle Power Magazine from October 1956 documented that for the twenty five year period, **Mac beat 4,000 opponents arm wrestling without a loss**!

A 1986 Ironman magazine article by Vic Boff describes how Mac was 6'1.5" tall, weighted between 300 and 325 lbs, with a 20"neck and had 19.5" arms. A 1950 article written by Mac himself explains how he built his massive arm strength with the Heavy Barbell curl. In this article, Mac passionately describes men of that era who excelled at the curl and had the corresponding arm development to prove it.

Mac finishes the article on the curl with detailed descriptions of how he trained for massive arm power. "The handling and use of **block weights** and **kettlebells** as accessories to your Barbell training will improve your forearm and grip strength to match that of tremendous upper arm flexion and increase your ultimate in curling." Mr Bachelor proudly stated that he was able to curl a 75 lb kettlebell with each arm by holding the bell with only his middle finger as well as being able to one arm curl a 90 lb dumbbell in the thumb up position. "With practice it is possible to stop the weight at any given point and rotate the wrist if the arm has been trained properly as a unit."

Mac described a favorite way to train his arm power: Sit in a chair with a 100lb dumbbell between your feet, with the collars almost touching opposite ankles, palm of the hand gripping facing the body start, disengaged hand resting on the corresponding knee, body bent over. Then spin the dumbell on the floor supinating the hand until palm is forward (curl position). At this instance, curl to the shoulder as you sit up and press strongly with the disengaged hand on the corresponding knee. The original momentum from the spin on the floor brings the bell easily to the shoulder at the completion as you sit upright.This exercise was apparently an awesome assistance exercise for arm wrestling prowess.

Mac was not just a one trick pony regarding his physical cultural pursuits with arm strength.

He possessed full body power that he increased by training in his well stocked home gym, performing Powerlifting based **workouts twice per week- doing speed squats cold with 350lbs for 20 reps without wraps or a belt!**

This type of whole body power enabled Mac to achieve the following strength achievements which were documented by strength historian Pete Vouno: shouldered a 700 to 800 lb telephone poll that was 40 feet long and walked with it for 300 feet at the Telephone Company in Los Angeles and another time he carried a 600 to 700lb small horse over 40 feet and then up a 16 ladder.

Mac's pinch gripping strength was unparalleled, walking distance with thick plates pinch gripped that others could not lift off the ground- such as waking 30 feet with pinching an 80lb plate in each hand that was 1.5" thick.

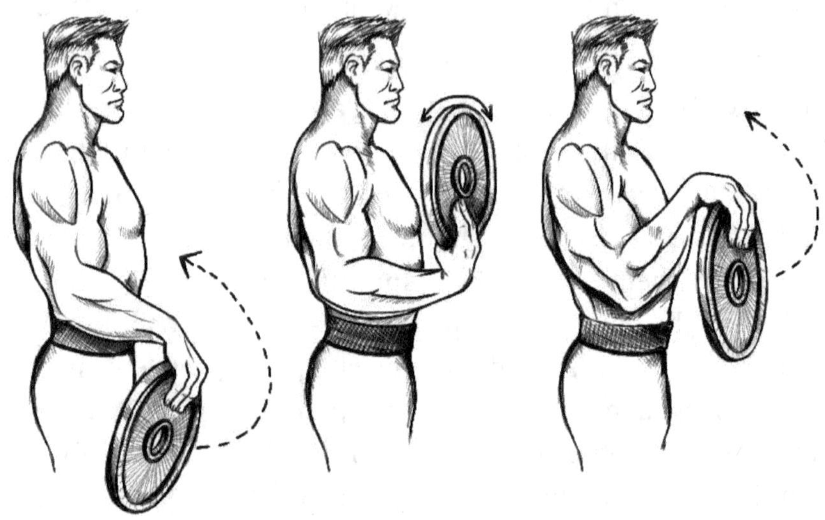

Mac penned a 1957 Muscle Builder article specifically on how he built he **world class wrist strength**, focusing on 3 exercises. According to Mac these three exercises will "add inches of muscle to your forearm, power pack your wrist with giant tendons and double the present power of your grip." The first exercise requires that you hold a weight plate at shoulder height, with 4 fingers on one side, the top of the plate and the thumb underneath the plate. With your arm locked out, raise the plate as far as you can upwards and then slowly lower it back to parallel to the ground. Do as many reps as you can strictly until you feel a deep ache in your forearm. The second exercise calls for the lifter to hold a weight plate at your side with a bent arm, 90 degrees from the floor. With 4 fingers on one side of the plate and thumb on the other side- also known as a pinch grip, rotate your hand as far as you can to the left, then to the right while holding the pinch grip as long as possible. Keep the palm of your hand and therefore the plate facing up. You can do this simultaneously with both arms or one at a time to really overload your hands and wrists.The third exercise is just to repeat the 2nd exercise but have the plate facing down for the entire pinch grip. With both #2 and 3, a circular motion with the plate really builds the wrist.

Mac suggests that the trainee start with a light weight plate such as 5 or 10 lbs. He uses a 25lbs plate.

Willis Reed, a powerfully built man and gym owner in Hollywood, California, wrote an article about Mac Bachelor. Reed described how athletic Bachelor was, able to do handstand push-ups at 325 lbs bodyweight, while playing competitive basketball and wrestling. Willis documents Mac's best lifts as a 220 lb curl, 500lb squat, 400 lb bench press, a 700lb deadlift, and a 275lb military press with heels together- which ranked him at that time as one of the strongest men who ever lived.

Mac made his living as a bartender in one of the most popular bars in Los Angeles, with a magnetic personality that drew professionals for every walk of life who were drawn to Mac and his memorable conversational abilities. Like a lot of big strongmen, Mac died later in life while suffering from numerous health ailments in 1986 – 30 years after he had been the world wrist wrestling champion of the world. I prefer to reflect on all Mac's strength accomplishments then to dwell on his demise which proved he was a mortal.

Jon Cole Strength Savage

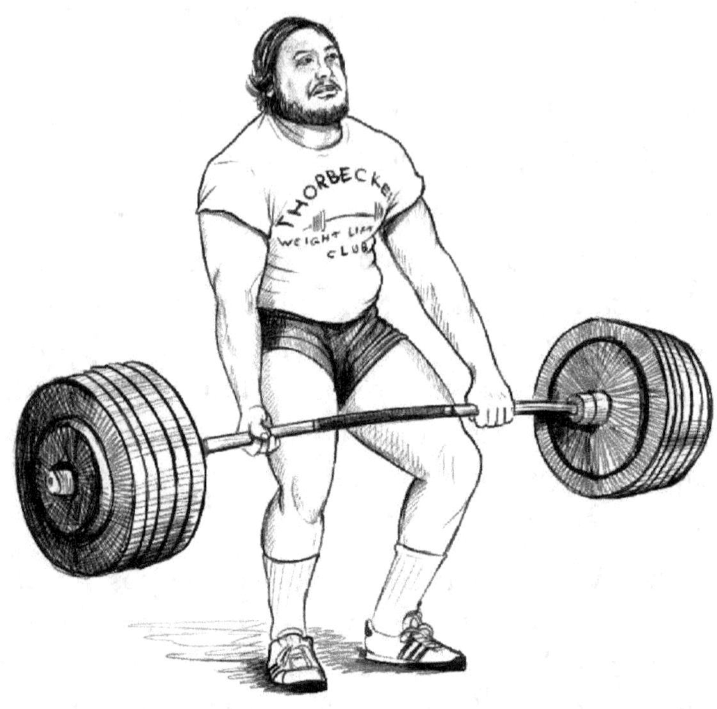

Jon Cole is still revered by hard core strength training practitioners the world over for the feats he accomplished almost 50 years ago. Jon held the all time super-total record for over a quarter of a century, with the highest official combined powerlifting and Olympic lifting totals. Jon weighed 282 when he did his best official lifts and held the super- total record until it was broken by 400lb Marc Henry. Although Louie Simmons and Westside Barbell get much credit for the popularization of the conjugate or concurrent system of training, Cole used that system in the late 1960s to build his incredible strength, without naming it conjugate.

I have been fortunate enough to interview Jon's long time training partner, Marv Allen, as well as others who trained with Jon or saw him train such as Brick Darrow and Mike Civalier. Bruce Wilhelm wrote an excellent article about Jon for Milo and Herb

Glossenbrenner also documented Jon and his training philosophy in Powerlifting USA Magazine.

Herb gave me the video footage of the 1972 Arizona State Powerlifting Meet at which Jon hit the first official 900lb squat and also benched 580, with a close miss at 600lbs – this footage appears on my Instagram as well as my YouTube Channel, Paul L.

Ron Fernando was a fabulous training writer for Powerlifting USA Magazine and was Arizona based during Cole's peak years so he was able to correspond with Jon and document their conversations. Jon detailed his training to Ron, and it is exactly how Wilhelm and Ken Leistner described hearing it also from Jon.

Ron Fernando and Dr. Ken Leistner both documented what Jon told them in published material, as well as Bruce Wilhelm who trained with Jon at his peak and can be seen spotting in the footage of Jon's 900lb squat. All three of these esteemed strength scribes details how Jon would bench and squat in the same workout and then do arm work. Jon preferred to bench press twice per week one week with one incline bench workout between the regular bench workouts. One bench workout would be a 5 X 5 with medium weight and the other workout would be 5 sets of 3 reps heavy. The incline workout would be a 5 X 5 between the two bench press workouts.

The next week there would two incline bench workouts, one heavy with 5 sets of 3 and one medium with 5 sets of 5 reps. In between those two workouts would be a regular bench press workout that was 5 sets of 3 reps for heavy sets.

On days he did flat bench work, his primary assistance exercise would be standing tricep extensions. On the day he did incline bench sets, he would do lying tricep extensions on a flat bench. Jon would do lots of standing barbell curls on days that he did a tricep exercise. For his arm work, Jon preferred 5 sets of 8 repetitions. Jon would alternate doing curls first in the workout before tricep extensions. The next week, he would do tricep extensions first before curls.

Jon would deadlift heavy once every two weeks according to Ron Fernando, alternating with the Olympic lifts done the following week. I interviewed Marv Allen in 2005. Marv was Jon's long term training partner in the 1970s and he said Jon would deadlift once per week. The day Jon would deadlift he would not squat that day. Jon loved back squats, but he would also do 5 sets of 3 front squats the workout before he would deadlift. Analysis of this exercise selection and placement indicates to me that Jon wanted his back to be rested and ready for the deadlift workout, so he would give it a break with front squats before deadlifting, as front squats would not load his back as heavy as regular squats.

In talking with Brick Darrow, he said Jon would tell him they needed to finish a workout with fingers and toes- which meant forearm work and calf work. One only needs to look at the image of Jon on the December 1994 Powerlifting USA to realize he had 22" arms at approximately 250 lbs bodyweight. Jon's calf routine was 6 sets of 20 reps with 2 sets of toes pointed in, 2 sets pointed out, and two sets of feet straight calf raises. Brick, who has run a Powerlifting gym for over 50 years has seen many powerlifting legends, but he says Jon was

"a true freak of nature" with a size 10 shoe, so he was no genetic monster. He said Jon would add cans of tuna fish to casseroles he would eat in an effort to bulk up to break the all time total record on multiple occasions. At the time of Jon's 6 plus hour powerlifitng workouts, Jon would drink a can of Nutrament every hour to fuel his body.

There are reports online at the Ironmind Forum that Jon once did a dip with 500lbs attached to his body for a single rep. I have read reports from famous powerlifter Gus Resthwich that he saw Jon do behind the neck presses with 285lbs as well as smoking a universal forearm wrist roller at its highest setting with blazing speed. When I posted about Jon on my Instagram recently, a person posted that he used to see Jon riding his bicycle on University Avenue in Tempe, going between Thorbecke's and the gym at ASU. Jon, who had an intense personality by all accounts, would train for 6 to 8 hours per day, twice a week on Tuesday and Friday. Multiple training locations and stimulations in the same workout is an example of the conjugate system of training.

Jon, who had a rivalry with Paul Anderson in the pages of Muscular Development, followed Paul's lead by getting as strong as possible on the powerlifts as well as the incline bench, and this carried over to Olympic lift success. According to interviews with Jon, by Herb Glossenbrenner and Bruce Wilhelm, Jon preferred to train the powerlifts instead of the three Olympic lifts of the day. Today's lifters could take much from Jon's philosophy of handling the most weight in the traditional powerlifts, while still doing frequent muscle building workouts for his arms and shoulders with inclines and upright rows. I cannot find any reference as to what, if any, direct lat and upper back Jon did in addition to deadlifts, cleans, and upright rows. One look at Jon's physique told you that his body had no weaknesses.

There are many lessons to be learned from studying Jon's training and performances. Jon alternated heavy 5 sets of 3 reps training loads for a lift, with 5 sets of 5 rep workouts described as medium. Arms were worked twice per week with direct tricep and bicep work.

John Kuc

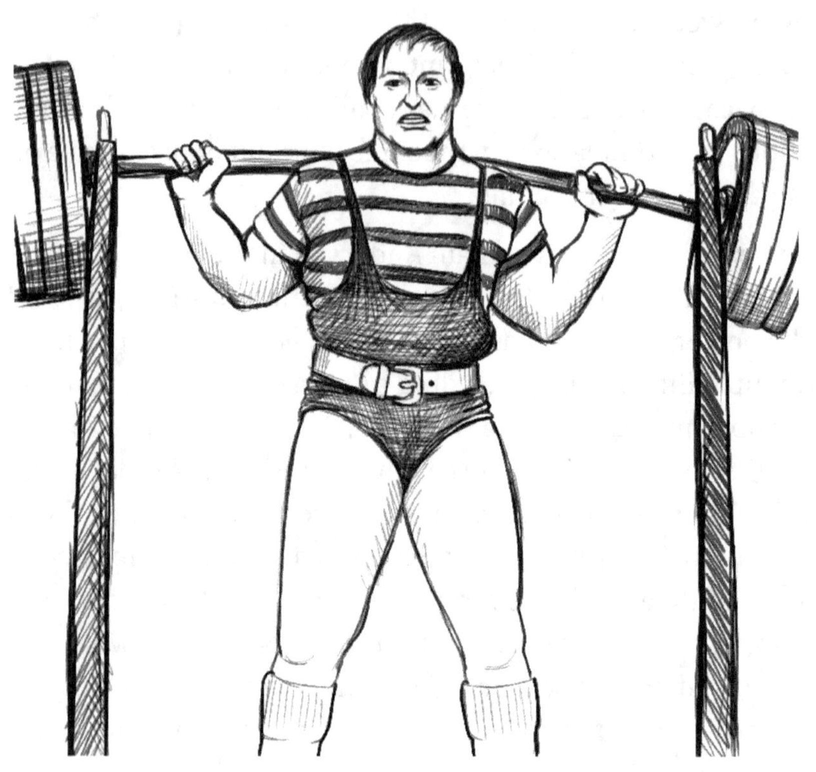

My fellow **Neckberg.com devotees, I wo**uld like to give you the gift of information that has been shared with me by some of the best lifters of all time-solely in the spirit of the Christmas/New Year season. Starting off, I would suggest any serious strength athlete obtain a copy of John Kuc's Kuc speaks on Powerlifting. This book has it all as far as training wisdom, of which I will share some gold that has worked for me. First, to maintain a strong lower back, do leg raises on the floor for a top set of high reps. John would do sets of 75 reps, had abs you could see through his singlet and conventionally pulled 870 at 242 in 1979, a world record that stood for over 30 years. For variety, you can occasionally do the leg raises on a grade like I do on my driveway. That angle really tractions my lower back and keeps it healthy.

Kuc provides a full 3 month pre-contest training journal with every set, rep, and exercise he did in building up to a world championship win. Two of Kuc's stalwart assistance exercises were lat pull downs and seated cable rows for 4 sets of 10 reps each with pretty moderate weights as compared to todays selectorized machines, but I have seen pictures of John's Pennsylvania based training lair and he worked with good old York plates that weighed their American made face value.

Kuc describes that aftermath of a deadlift workout, specifically that if your body does not ache and you were not exhausted after a deadlift session- then you wasted your fucking time. Reading Kuc's description of the effort needed to be a world class deadlifter always makes the hair on the back of my neck stand up.

For back health, I have always hung from a pull up bar for up to a minute or two. Kuc recommends hanging, but I have known about it approximately 15 years before I read Kuc's book when I had to hang to pass LAPD's physical test in the summer of 1991. Once I built up to over 2 minutes straight of hanging, my shoulders were bullet proof for the next decade. My favorite TV show is College Gameday and a recent video segment on Alabama's half a million dollar per year strength coach Scott Corcoran showed him making his football players/future millionaires hang from power racks for time. Those are primarily future NFL stars so I would say they are on to something. From 2004 to 2006, I trained with Josh Bryant while we prepped for the Atlantis Strongest Man in the U.S., with one of the events being a weighted pull up with a parallel grip. Josh won the whole show and did a pull up with 120lbs chained to his waist. I was able to do a pull-up with 75lbs attached to my waist, while I weighed 275lbs. My shoulders have never been stronger and due to the fact Josh military pressed 445 at that contest, I would say the same for him.

Another way in which I used to hang in training was when I was preparing to compete in the farmers walk. We would train in the street in front of the Freak Factory in Downey, California for various distances and with different weights per hand on one weekend day. Following event training my feet would ache and need rest for days, but my grip would be recovered by mid week. What we would do is hang from the power rack with a parallel grip to mimic the farmers walk but with heavy jump stretch bands over our shoulders that were attached to the base of the rack. The bands provided a great deal of resistance without placing more wear and tear on my lower body. I have seen a YouTube video of Donnie Thompson, a strength genius, who would traction his shoulders by placing heavy bands over his shoulders then lifting his arm to grab another band that was attached over head so he had bands pulling his shoulders in opposite directions simultaneously- yes!

Speaking of shoulder health, let's talk about what we used to do at Yorba Barbell to let our shoulders heal and re-build following the Powerlifting season of meets such as the California States in April, the Senior Nationals in July, and a fall meet in October or November- such as the old Ironman meet in Northern California. After two balls to the wall meet peaking cycles in the spring and fall, our shoulders needed a break from benching, especially many reps with bands attached. Westside Barbell had posted pictures of pro bodybuilder Mike Francois training at Westside and doing power rack military presses. Another Westside published article described how their top benchers at that time such as Joe McCoy and Kenny Patterson would do seated military presses with their upper backs braced.

These type of workouts were a welcome change from long ass bench shirt workouts where you might have done 8 total reps/ attempts in 2 hours as you took bench shirts on and off. What a waste of time! We would do either full range of motion military presses from the power rack cups and if someone was really tore up with inflammation from heavy benching all fall, then we might do partial over head presses from some power rack pins, ala Anthony Ditillo.

These workouts were also fun to do around the holidays because there was no pressure to hit pre-meet goals and every week your shoulders felt better doing these. Years later, when my good friend Mike Martin got to train with strength legend Jessie Kellum, Mike was told of the importance of doing your military presses the day after your heavy bench work. Mike has been able to bench over 400 lbs raw for 30 years so I would say he is on to something.

Have you walked the cooler aisle at your local convenience store lately? Enough energy drinks to choose from? Ever research pre-workout powders/concoctions at your local supplement store? I was fortunate enough to have trained in the 90s with Ultimate Orange, so you may understand why I am not impressed with today's energy supplements. I advise you to follow the lead of Paul Anderson by beginning any training session by hanging upside down so that blood can rush to the head in order to fuel the brain naturally. Following that, train your neck in all four directions so your neck holds up and your CNS lights up. If you have seen Westside Vs the World you know that Louie wished he had trained his neck more as now neck damage causes him to black out under load. In addition to neck, you can do other small muscle groups to wake up before your main training-provided whatever you do does not limit what you can lift on your main movements for the session.

There is nothing like hearing 'Twas the Night Before Christmas read by a powerful voice. For us lifters the closest thing we have is Donnie Thompson's Instagram which is a very informative and introspective by a man who dedicated his life to hitting the biggest all time total, all while not taking his internet persona too serious. For a harsher, yet brilliant look at the mind of one of the hardest powerlifters of all time, Greg Panora's Instagram is not to be missed. Greg, fellow Mass-hole, has been to hell and back to be the best of his time and he is a throat punch at a picnic to all the mainstream people who think they take Powerlifting serious. When the kids are in the car for those long trips over the holidays, Dave Tate's Elite FTS Table Talk podcasts are great as is any content from Barbell Logic is great stuff. You never really get past the basics in heavy lifting if you want to be great, plus Matt Reynolds has elite strength credentials and will provide value to any level of strength athlete with his intelligent insight.

Last but not least is all of the free content from Neckberg.com. I know this time of year, Sascha gives strength to the community and lifters an opportunity to learn about successful strength training methods as well as legends of the physical culture realm. Now that is the spirit. Enjoy your holidays all and prep your self for a great new year.

Become a Powerlifter

My journey in powerlifting and strength sports, what I would do differently and what I would not change.

2022 marks the 36th anniversary of my first powerlifting contest, when a non sanctioned meet was contested at the YMCA I trained at in West Roxbury, Massachusetts. I always wanted to be a big and strong person as soon as I began junior high school in 7th grade. I began lifting weights on my own in high school with one of those 110lb Sears weight set and bench press in my garage. Once high school began, I discovered lifting weights for football, with an emphasis on the bench press and some squatting- but not powerlifting.

A small, unsanctioned powerlifting meet was contested at the local YMCA I was training at. I squatted 315, benched 260 and deadlifted 405 in my first meet, after training for 6 weeks following the end of my high school football career. I weighed about 220, and at 6'2" Sknew I had the desire and the frame to build muscle and pursue powerlifting with everything I had.

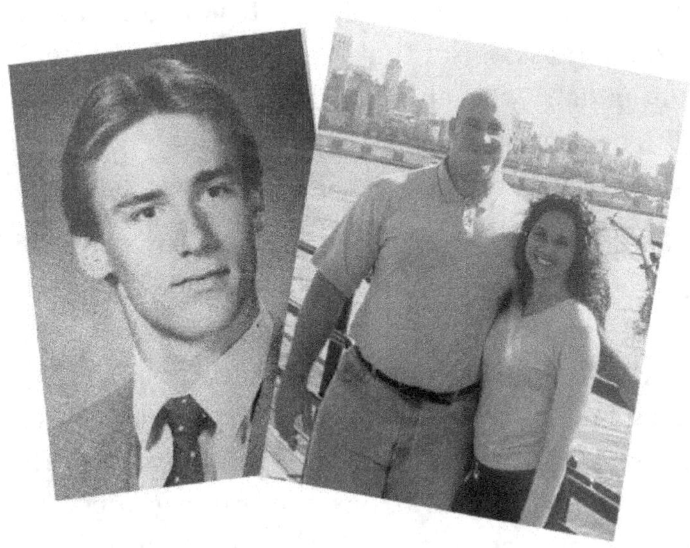

I grew from that 17 year old who totaled 980 to a man who would weigh as much as 325 and squat 810 bench press 534 and deadlift 750 for a total of 2094 in the official lifts. I did a lot of things right, but I also made many mistakes. If I had to do it all over again, I would advise a 17 year old male to do the following:

1. Find dedicated training partners. I am on my 5th or 6th generation of training partners since I began training. I prioritized my education, career, and family at the appropriate times in my life. I had periods of time when I did not have training partners because of my aforementioned priorities. When I had regular training partners, I made the most training and competitive progress. I say this after analyzing my 30 plus year competitive career.

2. Include some aerobic training for three or four sessions per week. Strength cardio is best such as medley style work of farmers walks and dragging or yoke and sled work. Use moderate weight and move dynamically to increase your heart rate and build your cardio respiratory system.

3. Pay better attention to nutrition. Stan Efferding's vertical diet is a great program to follow- steak and rice with salt being the cornerstone of a strength athlete's fuel. I ate a large amount of dairy, carbohydrates and protein powder in my quest to become as big and strong as possible. I should have focused on nutrient dense meats such as beef and buffalo.

4. Incorporate strongman training into my powerlifting program. The strongest athletes in the world when I started lifting were powerlifters. There were no strongman contests in the U.S. Today you can see that men such as Zydrunas Savickas, Eddie Hall, Brian Shaw and Thor Bjornsson are the strongest dead lifters and lot pressers in the world. They do lots of powerlifting and strongman training to become the ultimate hybrid strength athletes. Their YouTube videos show incredible weights being lifted in the powerlifts,

rowing movements,incline presses, smith machine presses, arm work, and leg pressing movements.

5. I would have traveled more to different training crews once I was an elite lifter. I had been invited to Westside Barbell on a few occasions and have not gone yet.

6. Read all you can about training from the experts. **Louie Simmons**, Josh Bryant and Matt Wenning produce great material. Find Dr. Ken Leistners writings from Milo or his newsletter from the 80s, the Steel Tip. Buy John McCallum's the Keys to Progress. Build your body while you are a teenager with hypertrophy work as they call it now.

   Bill Kazmaier had amazing programs of how to build muscular bulk and power, as did Anthony Ditillo. I followed and still do study these experts. Push up your 20 rep squat. I got mine to 315 for 20, and squatted 600 for 1 at 21. I should have pushed my 20 rep squat to at least 100 lbs over my weight of 240 for 20. High rep squatting builds your whole body like nothing else.

7. Play sports when you are a teenager and in high school. The group setting with peers will teach you how to push yourself and you will meet training partners you may have for life. Today, many high school weight rooms have incredible facility that are just for the athletes so take advantage. I would also suggest you take a martial art to build your fitness base. I took American style TaeKwondo and today Jiu Jitsu is popular. The flexibility, endurance, cardio capability and mental toughness gained from the arts cannot be replicated.

8. I used to travel to local gyms all over New England when I was young. I saw the Ultimate Warrior do a set of Upright Rows with 315 for a set of 10. It was impressive to say the least! Today, a young lifter can see famous athletes from around the world perform their workouts on social media.

You can ask them questions and interact with them. My close friend Josh Bryant has amazing content as Jailhousestrong on YouTube and Instagram. Josh trained Brian Shaw during the pandemic and Brian shared these training sessions on YouTube! I just watched Brian's latest YouTube video of his first training session of 2022, now under the guidance of Joe Kenn, long time strength coach from College Football and the NFL.

9. Research old school workouts of the greats in the Iron Game as profiled on Neckberg.com.

10. Find a Doctor who supports your goals and dreams as a strength athlete. I had amazing doctors in California, one in Texas and now in Arizona. You will never get strong if you are not healthy. As I write this, we are entering the second year of the pandemic. I have friends who have recovered easily from the virus- as they are strong and health conscious. Never settle for anyone who does not support you getting as strong as you can be in a safe and healthy manner. My doctors are always amazed by my laboratory work after 40 years of lifting. I tell them all the time what to do. Whether they listen is up to them.

How My Deadlift Increased from 405 to 600+ IN FOUR YEARS

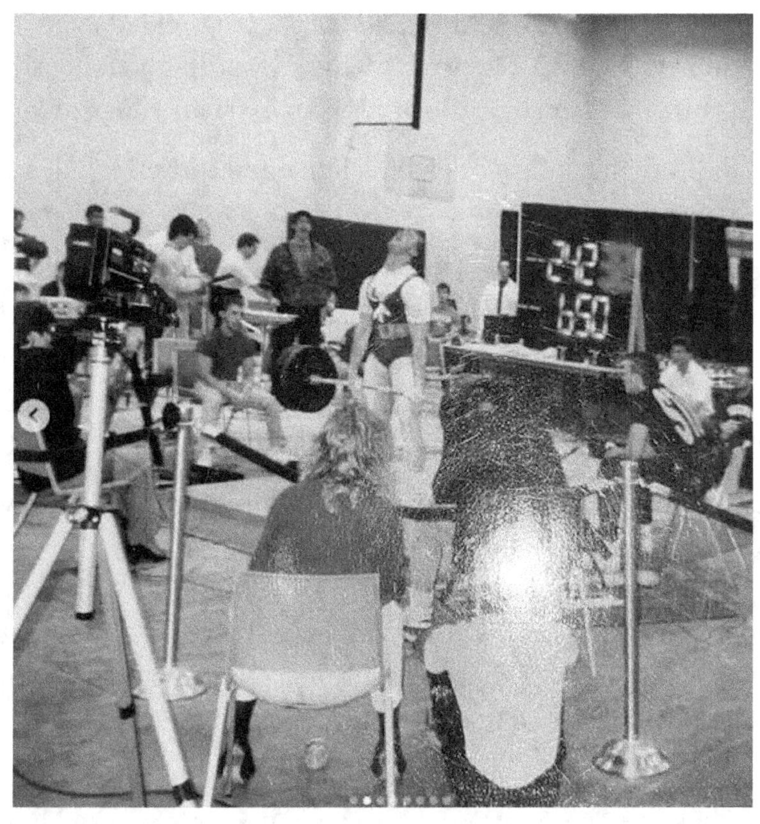

I lifted weights when began playing high school football in 1983. I played my last HS game, as the starting right guard, on Thanksgiving Day 1985, as my Boston Latin Wolfpack defeated Boston English in the game's 99th meeting. While playing football, my best bench was 250lbs and my squat was 275 for 5. I never deadlifted while playing football. As soon as football ended, I began training at the local YMCA and noticed a posted flyer for a powerlifting meet to be held at the gym on January 11, 1986. I did the meet with two of my buddies and I squatted 315 benched 260 and deadlifted 405- the first time I tried it.

I trained my deadlift very traditionally back then, based upon Powerlifting USA Magazine articles by John Kuc, Fred Hatfield and Dr. Ken Leistner. I would deadlift up to a heavy set of 5 reps on the deadlift after my lighter, usually high bar squat workout. By October of 1986, I pulled 550 in a meet having pulled every week since January. In 1987, I injured my back by stupidly doing stiff leg deadlifts off a flat bench press- getting an extreme range of motion.

To rehabilitate this injury, I read Bill Starr and Dr Ken articles about lower back rehabilitation.

The rehab took all summer, coupled with an arduous physical labor job, took a while to heal my back. As 1987 was coming to a close, my back was better so I began to train hard for the USA Teenage East Coast Open held in Gaithersburg, Maryland, my last meet as a teenager. I over trained my deadlift and pulled 560, missing 600.

In the summer of 1988, I finally pulled 600lbs, but I had not lived up to my personal goals. I began researching training and had some great, more experienced partners who gave me advice. I settled on a low repetition program after straining something in my back trying to rep 500 pounds for ten reps. My posterior chain was strong yet I learned that I would strain ligaments if I tried for too many repetitions – over 5, in the deadlift.

By 1989, I knew that working up to a heavy triple worked best for me. In 1990, I was training hard and in good shape, having tripled 590 in the deadlift, ten days before the USPF Region 1 Championships in New Hampshire on February 10th- the same day Buster Douglas knocked out Mike Tyson. I won the Junior (Under 23) Men's Open Division with lifts of 589 359 639. Six weeks later, I entered the 1990 ADFPA Collegiate National Powerlifting Championships at Virginia Tech University.

I squatted 600 benched 365 and deadlifted 650lbs at 237lbs. I came in 3rd overall in total and the deadlift was a Collegiate and American national record, beating the record of Randal McDaniel who went on to the NFL Hall of Fame.

My training for the deadlift back then was simple in that I focused on heavy triple once per week. I would pull on Wednesdays after light high bar squats. Bent over rows were my only assistance work, done for reps of 5 with a belt.

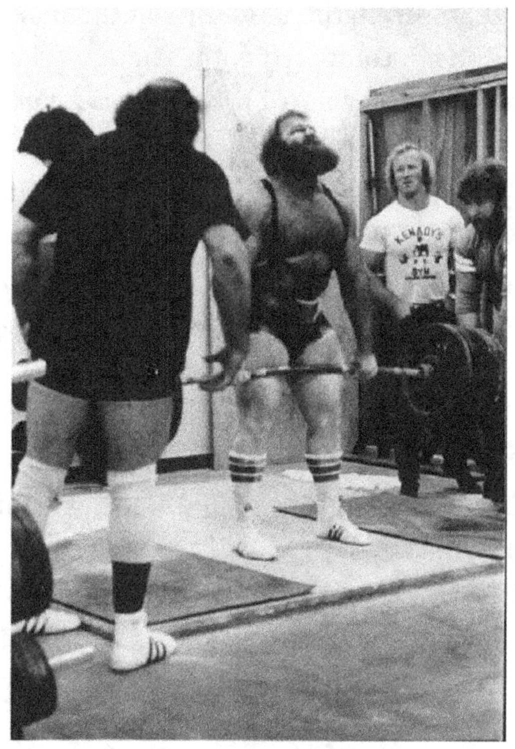

PHOTO COURTESY SHARAYAH JOHNSON

In 1986 Doyle Kenady, multiple time world powerlifting champion broke the deadlift all time world record with 903. He tried a 920 and just missed. He also squatted 847 and benched 547 for a 2293 total. He just missed a 887 squat that day. After this performance, the great Fred Hatfield wrote articles that detailed how leading up to the meet, they trained together and Doyle did an 895 triple in the deadlift. That is where I realized triples suited me well as an intermediate puller.

During the same time period, my official squat went from 315 to 615. I followed a typical progressive overload style most of the time when I was preparing for a meet, with 3 weeks of 5 reps, 3 weeks of triples, 3 weeks f doubles, and two weeks of singles, peaking at the meet in 12 weeks. In the offseason, I followed Dr. Squat's high bar program with lots of close stance with a belt only for sets of 8 reps with as much weight as possible with good form. I am 6'2" with a long back, so squats strengthen my conventional deadlift- the only form of deadlift I have competed with. There were training blocks during this time period where I would do Dr Ken Leistner high repetition squat sets to build muscle and mental toughness. The best set I ever did was 315lbs for 20 repetitions with a belt at 240lbs bodyweight- not too impressive as my cardio was not great.

I did not do much abdominal work in the gym, but for the first two years of this period of time, I studied American Style Taekwondo. This training was intense stretching as well as some abdominal training to support kicking power. I am sure this regime helped me stay injury free and led to my general physical preparedness, a term I would not hear until 7 years later, being very high.

How I would train my 17 year old self, using the training principles of Iron legends Bill Kazmaier, Jon Cole and Pat Casey.

If I were to go back to the beginning of my powerlifting career, I would focus on a Jon Cole based cycle for my competitive powerlifting training, Bill Kazmaier style training for muscular hypertrophy building in the off season and Pat Casey for bench press and shoulder specialization as my upper body always lagged behind my lower body development in my younger years of training.

Jon Cole's training was focused on squats, bench presses and deadlifts. He would also train the incline press, the upright row, the front squat, calf raises along with tricep presses and barbell curls. Although Jon competed at a National level in Olympic weightlifting, he built his strength through the powerlifts as well as the aforementioned assistance exercises. Jon held the all time super total record of the highest official combined powerlifting and Olympic lifting total for over 25 years! Cole did his best lifts at no more than 282 lbs, while his super total record was finally broken by 400lb Mark Henry.

I have studied Jon's career, read experts reports such as former training partner Bruce Wilhelm, Dr Ken Leistner, Ron Fernando and Herb Glossenbrenner- I have also got to interview those who trained with Jon such as Brick Darrow, Mike Civalier, Marv Allen and Dave Keaggy. Due to having an understanding of how Jon trained as well as the results he obtained, I feel his system is a great way for a beginning powerlifter to train. The emphasis on sets of 5 or 3 repetitions in the competitive lifts as well as higher reps in his preferred assistance work would build strength and muscle mass while also correctly focusing on the progressive overload that is the key to success in any weight sport.

When I began Powerlifting training at 17, I followed the information in the magazines of the day, with much great information coming from Fred Hatfield's published works in Powerlifting USA and Muscle and Fitness Magazines. Of course, I overtrained as an enthusiastic youth, but never suffered any long term injury and I built a base that allowed my official total to go from 980 to 1600 as a drug free 21 year old, wearing single ply gear. I got lots right in my training, but if I had known about Cole's system/philosophy of training I would have done better.

Cole was an athlete through out his life and as a young man, I had goals of getting into a law enforcement career- so I did not need to become a superheavy weight powerlifter at that stage of my life. I needed to become stronger while still maintaining an athletic and functional physique. I know that following his illustrious strength competition days, Jon loved to ride a bicycle. One of my recent posts on Instagram about Jon has a post underneath it from a former student who used to see Jon riding his bike in Tempe between ASU and Thorbeckes gym. Jon would train for long workouts at his peak- up to 6 hours per session!, but later in life it is apparent that he would spread his workouts out amongst different locations.

Jon finished his powerlifting career in the 242lb class, lifting world class weights at the

Hawaiian Invitational. Similar to Bill Kazmaier, who lifted his greatest powerlifting lifts at 340lbs, he reduced to 320 to dominate the major strongman contests of his time. Pat Casey as well got in the best aesthetic shape of his career after he finished his powerlifting career, as evidenced by a famous shot of Pat posing at Muscle Beach in the late 1960s. This would be a model for my later strength career, but I am getting ahead of myself.

Pat Casey was a huge influence on powerlifters everywhere when he became the first man to total 2000lbs, squat 800 and bench press 600. Pat's upper body training sessions were also notoriously long. Pat also was featured in an article at the time where he detailed his shoulder specialization program to build lasting shoulders, a key foundation for powerlifting success as all three power lifts require considerable shoulder strength to perform well. Pat Casey was reportedly a huge fan of Jon Cole and would travel to Arizona to see Jon set some of his all time world record lifts. I know that Jon did a great deal of shoulder work as well because he was the second best Olympic lifter in the U.S. when the press was still contested.

Pat Casey's bench press and shoulder press specialization courses focused on heavy partial benches, pullover and presses, weighted dips, and incline dumbbells for very heavy weight as well as low repetitions.

Pat Casey's shoulder specialization program called for three days per week of overhead pressing with barbells or dumbbells, sometimes with one dumbbell at a time for the overload factor. Pat advised to do side laterals as well as handstand push-ups. Initially did alot of military presses when I began training in my basement at 14 and did not have a spotter- therefore the military press could be worked to failure safely. I did behind the neck presses as well. Once I began lifting at my high school with my football team, I emphasized the bench press far too much.

No discussion of shoulder strength and training can be had without examining the training of Bill Kazmaier. Kaz held numerous shoulder pressing records such as the log press world record in his time, as well as the record for pressing a pair of 155 lb dumbbells for 5 reps. Kaz authored 3 courses sold in the 80s, one about the squat/deadlift, one about the bench press, and the final one focused on increasing your muscular hypertrophy. Bill's course said that in order to build muscle mass, it was far better to sweat a lot than to urinate. Kaz said that a 1/8" an inch of muscle is far greater than a pound of fat. Kaz continued with his philosophy that in order to build the most muscle, a lifter needed to divorce themselves from the concept of lifting very low repetitions with long rest periods.

When Kaz was inducted into the International Sports Hall of Fame at the Arnold

Schwarzenegger Classic, he thanked iconic bodybuilder Bill Pearl for teaching him the keys to the inner universe- other wise known as Pearl's bodybuilding secrets and the meaning of physical culture. When I was a teenager, no strength athlete in the world received more media coverage in the Powerlifting and bodybuilding magazines as well as on television for powerlifting competitions and his World Strongest Man appearances. Going back to his ISHOF speech, Kazmaier is a strength decathlete- great at every strength sport he entered.

Kazmaier's training protocol was to do enormous amounts of training volume by higher repetitions such as 10 and higher number of sets of exercises to obtain the desired volume which built his unparalleled muscularity. I had extremely successful training cycles following Bill's off-season program of bench presses with wide and narrow grip, standing dumbbell presses, triceps pushes with an ez curl bar, and a huge amount of upper back and latissimus work. Squatting and deadlifting were done for reps of 8 to 10, with leg extensions, leg curls, and calf work in earnest. Kaz worked every body part to include abdominals with weighted

Roman chair sit-ups and side bends. Bill did not specify neck work, but he detailed an exhaustive amount of shrug work he did twice per week- at times doing as many as forty repetition with heavy barbell shrugs.

As far as my documented belief in Westside Barbell's conjugate style of training- I do believe that is best applied once a lifter has a strength base as well as the muscle mass to support future strength gains. Such foundational goals are best obtained via a Cole, Casey and Kazmaier hybrid training approach. They were trailblazers and all looked every bit the iconic strength and power legends they were through intelligent, hard work. They also contributed to society as Pat was a police officer and gym owner, while Jon and Bill were professional strength coaches in the collegiate and private sector. My goal was to be a successful powerlifter while having a law enforcement career which I was able to do for over 30 years.

My First Year of Westside Barbell Lower Back and Abdominal Training

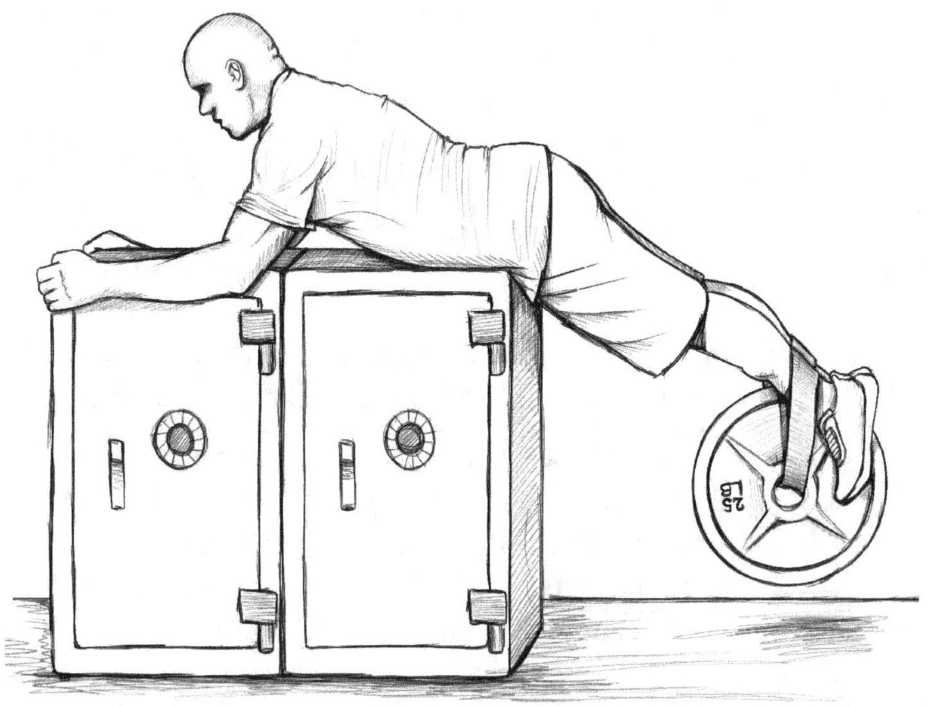

When I began training Westside style, I had very limited equipment options and a 1600lb total in 1994. One of the most important aspects of Westside Barbell System is the strengthening of your back. Louie Simmons agrees with the immortal Bill Kazmaier who said "a strong man has a strong back." I trained in a work office that would be converted to a workout space at night when the employees went home. A boom box and Louie's Powerlifting USA articles were my train partners for my first year of Westside training. The office belonged to my old delusional boss, who stocked it well when he wasn't binge eating Klondike's like a teenage girl. I had full access to an Ironmind Squat Stand, 700lbs in plates, PowerBlock dumbbells to 120lbs, a power bar and curl bench seat to squat to. With these Spartan resources I built a 633 lb squat and 672 deadlift, to go with a 424 bench I officially registered by the end of 1994.

No Reverse Hyper Machine, No Problem

When I began Westside, I realized I did not have access to a reverse hyper machine, the patented device that Louie instructed was essential for lower back strength and health. The first thing I did to address this was to take a traditional brown leather weight belt and cut it so that it could be slipped through the hole on a 25 lb plate and the buckle could be tightened around my ankles. With plates secured by my ankles, I would hop up onto a bank of 5 drawer safes and I was able to perform a reasonable facsimile of the reverse hyper movement. The weights would bang off the safes at the bottom of the movement but it did work alright given the situation.

The modified reverse hyper helped but I built my back strength by doing the following exercises. After my four weekly workouts, I would do Dimmel deadlifts, which were from the hang, with straps using 25% of my maximum deadlift. I would use between 135 to 185 for 2 sets of 20 reps in the movement, building up speed during the set- lowering the bar quickly to stretch my hamstrings and then returning to lockout explosively. I would rest 2 minutes between the sets. This resulted in my volume for my hamstrings being increased by 320 repetitions per month. Louie has said that elite sprinters would average 600 reps of hamstring work per month- so with the Dimmels and Dynamic Effort Squat and Deadlift work, as well as Max Effort lower body work, I was very close to 600 reps for my lower body per month. I would do these with 135 for 20 on upper body days, Max Effort and Dynamic Effort. On lower body days I would go with 185 for 20 reps.

After Dimmels, I would do abdominal work- specifically leg raises on upper body days and weighted sit up work on lower body workout sessions. Abdominal work was done for two or three hard sets of weighted resistance. Leg raises were often done with the reverse hyper belt on the ankles with weights attached.

Twice per week I would do side bends with the power block dumbbells for two sets of 20 reps per set with straps so that my grip was never an issue.

Janda style sit-ups were attacked on sit up day. I did these by jamming my toes under safe handles and getting my heels as close to my butt with my legs bent at 90 degrees. Then with a 25, 35 or 45 lbs plate behind my head, I would squeeze my torso off the floor and cramp the shit out of my abdominal wall.

For upper back I did bent over rows from the floor, with a power belt and straps. My goal was 3 sets of 5 reps with 50% of my deadlift. So 350 for a 700lb puller. These were not super strict nor were they cheated up. At the time, Dorian Yates was Mr. Olympia and was famous for bent over rows- yes sir, count me in.

That is the above program I did to put over 100 lbs on my powerlifting total in one year and burn off about ten pounds of pure fat that I had gained in error, before I began Westside. As Louie says, big ain't strong, strong is strong.

My First 3 Years of Westside Barbell Training

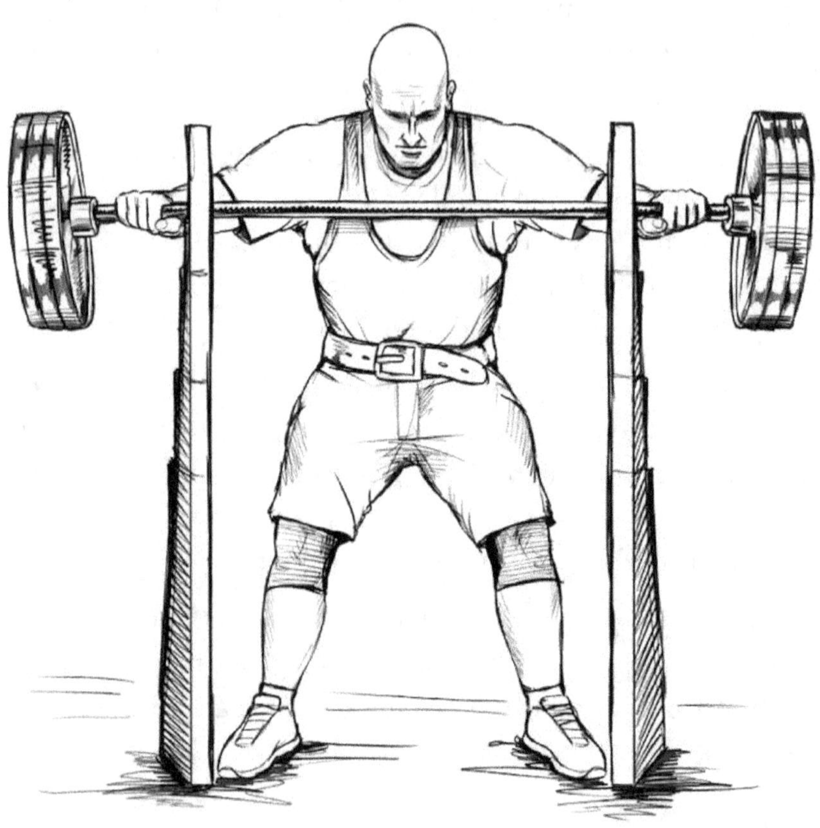

In approximately 1988 I first read about Louie Simmons and the Westside Barbell Club Ohio in issues of Powerlifting USA. I read anything I could get my hands on about getting stronger then, but I did not follow or apply any of the principles Louie discussed in those late eighties issues. I trained traditional linear periodization and my best lifts increased from 1250 to 1600 in four years, with a squat of 615, bench of 380 and deadlift of 650 in competition.

My then girlfriend had bought me the Westside Barbell tapes for Christmas 1993. As Louie Simmons has said many times, in the beginning all he had was a power rack, an AM FM radio, and the Powerlifting magazine articles of the time. I would train max effort bench with Powerhouse Gym in Chatsworth on Wednesdays to grab a spotter but no one in my life then was serious about training the squat or the deadlift. My boss at the time was in a serious midlife crisis mixed with delusional tendencies of which I was the benefactor because he purchased great equipment to train with at the office where we worked. I had 24/7 access to a Texas Power bar, 700lbs in plates, a squat stand, and a box to squat to.

As the youngest guy in the office by two decades, my co-workers would clear out by 5 to the life I know all too well now, kids activities or Home Depot runs for the latest Chinese plastic piece for my house that has surprisingly broke. I would have a snack, psyche up and set up the equipment in the 400 square foot main office. My workouts soon became ten minutes of terror as I would complete the dynamic effort box squat for ten or twelve doubles while I counted a minute between sets. As Louie has written, when you push your sets with little rest-you recruit dormant muscle fibers to get the job does. This lactic acid tolerance type training naturally raises your growth hormone level resulting in fat being burnt off and connective tissue being strengthened. I would squat to a below parallel preacher bench seat for my main dynamic effort squats with varied stances from close, medium, or wide.

At times I would do additional sets of squats with a very wide stance to a 10" milk crate for doubles. Remember I am 6'2" so this was quite the range of motion for my hips and entire posterior chain. Could that be why I am still training hard 25 years later? I followed Louie's recommendations the best I could with very limited equipment after my squats. I would do bent over good mornings, primarily for triples but I recall doing a single with 405 then. **Bent over rows were a staple as they are the 4th powerlift, the one assistance exercise that positively impacts the three competitive lifts.** Abs were done by hooking my feet under sturdy furniture and doing sit-ups of various widths and leg raises with and without weights. Reverse hyper were accomplished by placing weights on an old leather lifting belt that I had cut to fit the hole on an Olympic plate and doing the reps off of a bank of 5 drawer safes.

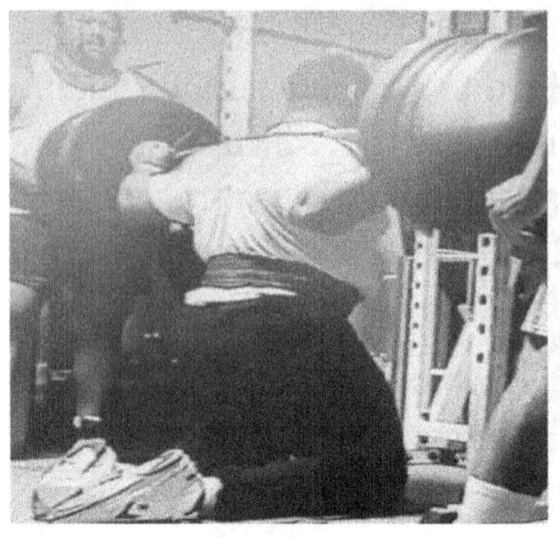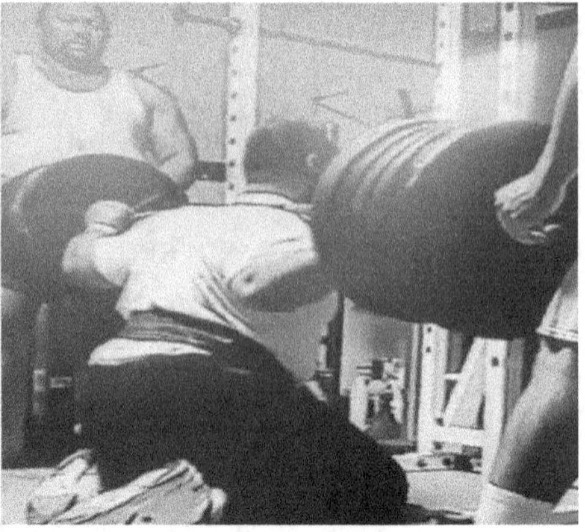

I followed Lou's advice to train Max Effort lower body with exercises I had never done before such as zercher squats, kneeling squats, pull throughs with a cable, and side bends. At this time in my lifting career, I had officially pulled 650 at 242 using traditional progressive overload training- whatever I could triple I could pull 60 pounds more in a meet. Louie's articles and tapes introduced to his dynamic deadlift method of doing sub maximal singles with very short rest periods. This 5 week cycle called for 15 singles at 65% of actual max, 70% for 12 singles, 75% for 10 singles, 80% for 8 singles, and 85% for 6 singles. On the 6th week I would pull a either a training max or a do a meet. If no meets in sight you could deload- a concept I never knew of until the 2000s.

For my benching I would do the dynamic effort workout using 65 % of my actual raw max. Bands and chains were not known to me at that time. Lou schooled me on **Dicks presses, Williams' front plate raises, triceps roll backs, floor pressing for reps,** and the importance of **dumbbell pressing from different angles** for hypertrophy work. Westside materials introduced me to **Bradford presses, chest supported row work**, and the need for **heavy hammer curls** that created forearms that allowed me to complete heavy powerlifts and later Strongman tasks. Louie also wrote about weighted push-ups for a record with different plates on your back.

In November of 1994 I decided to put my new training style to the test by doing the USPF Vandenberg AFB Open/Military Nationals. I weighed in at 260lbs and in the single ply gear of the day I went 633 407 677 for second place in the 275 lb class with my first official 1700lb total.

I met Steve Denison that day and he was a great resource who introduced me to my future training partners such as Art LaBare and Josh Bryant. My first few years in So Cal were not the lifting paradise I had envisioned when I left Massachusetts, but after 1994 my foundation was solidly laid and the best lifting years of my life were ahead.

Once I was convinced that Westside Style worked, I relocated to North Orange County for the best gym environment I could find in Southern California at the time. I had two training partners who trained with me and we all made great progress. I came in second to Steve at the 1995 California State Championships in the 275lb class with 661 413 705. Our workouts were fast, furious and productive. When I began Westside training, I immediately started doing conditioning exercises at the end of every training session. These conditioning exercises consisted of Dimel deadlifts at every session with up to 225lbs for two sets of twenty reps, often supersetted with abdominal work such as hanging leg raises or decline sit-ups with weight.

By 1996, I wanted to move up to a full Superheavy weight so I continued to train Westside style, my body just had acclimated to the intensity and pace of the training so I just added more quality food and protein and I grew bigger. I totaled my first 1800 and 1900 total that year. I came in 3rd with a 1934lb total of 733 457 744 at 296lbs at the WPC Can Am Championships in Las Vegas, Nevada. Westside lifters such as Chuck Vogelpohl, Tom Waddle, and Arnold Coleman were at the meet.

Westside Barbell takeaways from this article should be:

1. After 8 years of traditional progressive overload, the Conjugate style of training gave me a huge boost in competitive strength after following it for five years.

2. Dynamic effort training was a new concept for me but I followed Louie's guidelines and the %s and volume put me in great strength athlete shape. I lost body fat and built muscle mass.

3. Focusing on weak points in my lifts and muscular skeletal system worked very well for me. It created a fantastic foundation for me to compete at National Powerlifting Championships as well as high level strongman contests.

4. Without regular training partners like I left in Massachusetts, I was able to improve all on my own. Westside style training can be done entirely on your own with a few modifications and a power rack.

5. Training Conjugate was/is fun. As Louie says: You are always beating the weights so you don't walk around like your best friend died. There was no mental drudgery with training. People really believe in this system so you can find many pieces of information online about Westside training to inspire and instruct you.

6. Any video/dvd or webinar I have purchased from Westside Barbell has been worth it's weight in gold. The original 1993 video tapes for each 3 lifts were invaluable in my development as a powerlifter. I highly recommend any lifter in either raw or geared training, PED user or natural, to check these tapes out because they teach technique, special exercises and intensity!

7. As Louie Simmons says, everything works, but nothing works forever. Train hard and give the basic Westside template a chance and you will be convinced. Once

something stops working, research all the different exercises Louie has described and assess what will attack your weaknesses. As Louie says, do what you need to do, not what you like doing in the gym or what your training partner likes to do.

8. Read the free articles on Westside Barbell's website about the dynamic effort method, max effort method, and the repetition effort method.

9. I have followed Westside and Louie Simmons for almost 30 years. He has given so much of his time and advice for free. Buy his books, DVDs, and listen to his podcast because he continues to do the one thing that you need to do to be successful in life and the gym- analyze, apply, and evolve.

GPP training- its origins and implementation

General Physical Preparedness, or GPP, was a term I first learned while reading articles written by Louie Simmons in 1995 in Powerlifting USA and Milo magazines. Louie Simmons has justifiably been called The Godfather of Powerlifting as well as the Mad Monk of the sport. Based in Columbus Ohio his entire life, Louie lifted National and World Class weights in his twenties through his 60s!

After reading his book, the Iron Samurai, I learned that Louie had been a brick mason's assistant – called a block tender, since the age of 13. This manual labor job would have entailed carrying bricks, ladders, and other stone mason objects. Louie was also a great youth baseball player, once leading his city in home runs as a teen.

Louie described GPP as a degree of fitness which is an extension of absolute strength.Louie's

90s era recommendation to improve GPP was to use a sled dragging program. Over time, Louie has evolved from his recommendation of sled dragging to incorporate all types of strongman training in order to improve a strength athlete's GPP. Louie inspired me to keep my body in shape, to be a conditioned strength athlete capable of doing more work. The more work I could complete in the gym and recover from, the stronger I would become.

In the early 2000s, when I began training for and entering strongman contests, I determined that training the tire flip, farmers walk, yoke, dragging and stone lifting is the best way for a strength athlete to improve their GPP. The current onslaught of 900 and 1000lb deadlifts is proof that when a lifter is in better shape, that lifter can train harder, recover better, and make strength gains which were unprecedented less than 20 years ago. In 2003, there were only 9 men who had deadlifted over 900lbs officially, where recently in 2021, 6 Professional Strongman

Competitors pulled 1000 in the same Giants Live Contest! Eddie Hall and Thor both have pulled over 1100!

In a related point, Eddie came to strongman after being a high level competitive swimmer- and athletic base that is notoriously high in GPP. Thor was on Iceland's National Basketball team- again, a huge GPP base is built with the participation in high level competitive sports.

In the U.S., many strength athletes enter strength athletics after having been either a football player, wrestler, or any number of popular sports that teenagers are offered. These sports build a certain base of GPP that helps an athlete gain strength at a faster rate because they had a stronger foundation of fitness qualities before they began strength training.

These fitness qualities would be flexibility, aerobic capacity, inter muscular coordination, and endurance.

As for me, I loved to play outside when I was young. I ran, climbed trees, played tag, pickup ball games, rode a bike and a skateboard and walked/ran everywhere. You were told not to come home until it was dark and you played with your friends outside from sun up to sun down. In my early teens, I began playing organized sports such as little league baseball and volleyball. When I began high school, I started playing football- which was a great GPP builder with sprinting, form running, weight training, flexibility and hours on my feet at practice and games. As high school was ending, I began studying American style taekwondo, which introduced me to sparring, extreme flexibility and abdominal training. I began Powerlifting as soon as high school football ended so I was doing martial arts at the same time for a year.

I attribute my longevity in strength sports, with having done meets/contests for over 36 years, to my active upbringing and football training coupled with martial arts. In the 1940s, Bob Peoples held the world record in the deadlift with 700 lbs. Bob was a farmer- which is hard physical labor and a form of GPP.

Bob played football for a year at college in Tennessee, which also added to his GPP and power foundation.

Today, Dennis Cornelius, a top raw and drug tested powerlifter in the U.S. sets National records and also does jiu jitsu. The first powerlifter in the world to total 3,000 lbs,Donnie Thompson, had an extensive football career, playing arena league until training as a bodybuilder. Once Donny turned to powerlifting, he knew he needed to increase his GPP so that he would be able to set all timeworld records in powerlifting. What he did was become RKC certified in kettlebell training by Pavel Tsasouline.

As for how to program GPP training, Louie Simmons said he would use the 60% rule, meaning that he would go heavy on sled dragging for a distance of say 200 feet and then each of the next two days he would do 60% of the previous days weight for 200 feet. On the fourth day, he would program the lifter to do his heavy weight again and repeat the cycle. Louie Simmons has many free articles on his Westside Barbell Website regarding how to increase GPP.

The reality of improving your powerlifts by increasing your GPP is to pick an activity that builds your work capacity up and does not break you down for your main strength workouts. As long as you are setting lifting records and are healthy, keep doing as muchof whatever activity improves your overall fitness base.

From Westside to Strongman Competitor

I did my first powerlifting competition in 1986, and began training Westside Style in 1994. After two top 5 finishes at the Men's National Championships and a National Bench Press and Push Pull Championship, I got hurt at a local powerlifting meet and decided to rehabilitate my knee injury by engaging in strongman style training in January 2001. I had always known about the World Strongest Man Contest since I began powerlifting, but there were no opportunities for anyone to compete in strongman contests in the U.S. until the late 1990s. Milo Strength Journal and Powerlifting USA Magazine began reporting about strongman contests that were contested in the U.S., but they were held in Indiana and Texas, no where near California.

When I began rehabbing my knee, I met Kevin Kinzy, an accomplished Highland games athlete who had a background in martial arts as well as some local powerlifting meets. Kevin's training partner was professional strongman Charley Kaptur, all 6'10" 360lbs.

They immediately welcomed me into their training crew and I brought strength phenomena

Josh Bryant into the mix. I named our crew the Freak Factory and from 2001 through the 2000s, the crew had many strongman competition successes. There is a fantastic video on YouTube detailing the training of our group leading up to the 2004 California's Strongest Man Contest, which the Freak Factory instituted.

I just saw a clip on Power Athlete's Social Media where John Welbourne interviewed Fred Hatfield and Dr Squat said that he would have used strongman training to become the strongest he could have become if that style had been popular during his prime.

I agree with Dr Squat that strongman style training, combined with powerlift training is the secret to super human performance.

How we trained:

DE squat and dead workout on Tuesdays. We would primarily use a safety squat bar to save wear and tear on our shoulders. The safety squat bar with blue bands and 242lbs bar weight for 8 to 10 doubles to a 12" box. Dynamic deadlifts were done with 65 to 80% for singles with a minute rest between each single. Bent over rows/heaves were done with the ending set of deadlift weight. We would use a belt and straps and do 3 to 5 repetitions. Snatches were done occasionally, but for low reps and not more than 185 or 200lbs. We would attach strong bands (blue) to the bottom of the power rack and then pull the band over the each shoulder. This would pull the lifter towards the ground. Then we would hang by gripping with our hands on the chin up bar. We would do this for time to build our grip for the farmers walk. Our feet and lower body would not be recovered by Tuesday from Saturday's strongman events such as farmers walks, but our hands would be ready for grip work. This also tractioned our lower backs well.

Thick ez curl bar preacher work was next and it built strong arms for tire flips and stones, as well as Conan's wheel. Cable abs were done on a decline bench, facing away from the cable with a rope handle around the neck.

Medley work, was done for distance during the week, again on Tuesday following our DE Barbell work, with maybe 200 to 400 feet with 50 percent of the competition weight to be done on either Saturday or Sunday. Usually on Saturdays we would do our heavy strong man event day but for Boston in 2002, in an attempt for Kevin and myself to turn pro, we did Saturday and Sunday for 6 weeks up til the meet on 2/17.

My log clean sucked so I did DE work during the week- 65% for doubles- used the Westside Bench percentages. We did standing dumbbell clean then I presses with 2" thick handled dumbbells. 110lbs for 9 was my best with these dumbbells.

We had a 600lb tire that was used so the tread was worn. We used to attach our 20 lb chains to the inside of the tire so that the weight was up to 800lbs. We would flip tires at other locations often. Every tire is different. New tires feel different than old/used tires.

We trained three times per week usually with heavy event training on Saturday. We would warm up with deadlifts, my best was 585 for 6

and then we would flip our tire. Two or three trips of up to 100 feet with the tire loaded from 600 to 800lbs. At times we would begin the workout with farmers walk training. We would use up to 360lbs per hand for as far as we could go. We would each do 2 to 3 "runs" of as far as we could go with from 220 to 360lbs per hand. My competition weight was 300lbs per each hand. Professional competitor Charlie Kaptur had to use 360 per hand so I would use that at the end of my workout to over load the muscles that farmer walk.

Many times we would pull a semi-truck that Charley's company California construction owned. There is a picture of me on my Instagram pulling Charley's semi, which was loaded with a load of roofing tiles and a forklift. The truck scale said the load weighed 72,000 lbs and I was able to pull this 100 feet, twice in July 2001 on the first time I tried such a harness liftwhat a rush!!!!

Every few months we would deload and take the weekend off and play paintball as a crew. That was a lot of fun and kept us mobile. I only did strongman training events for a few years as my wife and I had twins to add to our 2 year old son in 2003, so I could not work full time and train strongman style any longer because I never could get enough sleep. Westside style Barbell training gave me a great base for strongman competition and training. I highly suggest you watch some of Brian Shaw's videos on YouTube and see how he combines the two styles of training to win the World Strongest Man Contest 4 times and be runner up this past year!

Emotional Intelligence Development and the serious lifter

Meathead, Muscle head, chunky trunk, hulk, gym rat, and other terms which could be viewed in either a positive or negative way have been used to describe those whose physical presence bears testimony to years spent under some serious iron.

Those with a habitual inclination towards exertion can be labeled many things by the members of general society who do not want to "get too big", as if such a state is possible. I am still waiting for the time I turn on "My 600lb Life" and it is referring to an individual so jacked that his body weight and the weights he routinely lifts are mind blowing. Call us serious gym disciples what you will but never call us dumb. There are thousands of studies that confirm the positive physical benefits of strength training, but what of any studies regarding the effects of intense training on the emotional well being of a person.

I am by no means a trained clinical psychologist or psychiatrist but I have spent a third of a century competing in high level strength athletics and I just completed a leadership course which focused on emotional intelligence as examined by the Harvard Business Review. After reflecting at length about the lessons taught in the course I will explain, in lifter-layman's terms how I know that strength athletics greatly increases an individual's emotional intelligence.

According to the Harvard Business Review the five components of emotional intelligence are self awareness, self regulation, motivation, empathy, and social skill. Let us take a closer look at each of these qualities and see how they are intertwined with gym performance.

Self awareness is critical if you are going to be successful in life period, let alone perform as a high level strength athlete. I have trained extensively with some of the strongest powerlifters in the U.S., men such as James Soroka, Art Labare, Josh Bryant and Mike Martin. These men all had one characteristic above all else in their personality, they knew exactly what they needed to do to perform at their best. The hallmarks of self awareness are self confidence melded with a realistic self assessment. None of my mentors and training mates were ever cocky, but they all oozed confidence in themselves in how they were training and how they lived their life in and out of the gym. Their enthusiasm was infectious and if they had a crappy day before hitting the gym, you would never know it as all that nonsense was checked at the door before we trained. The realistic self assessment allows a person to logically identify their weaknesses, figure out where they need to focus their training efforts for future improved performance, and ultimately allows the lifter to further boot their confidence because they realize that they alone have full control over their results. That's right, you own you!

Self regulation is a concept that has been important to lifters since I began lifting weights. In the 80s Muscle Fitness baron Joe Weider had a series of training rules called the Weider Principles, one of which was the instinctive principle. This principle basically instructed a lifter to train what they felt they needed to prioritize or to not train a certain muscle group or lift if it was not yet recovered. For the last ten years, auto regulation is a very popular term that is used to describe the training philosophy of many great strength athletes. My friend and

Powerlifting phenom Mike Tuchscherer is the founder of a successful company called Reactive Training Systems which is the most researched and practiced auto regulation training system in the world.

The Harvard Business definition of self regulation is the ability to control disruptive impulses. Think about that statement for a moment all of you lifters who attempt a max every time you are in the gym. How has that worked out for you? I know it is hard to resist the temptation to go too heavy all the time with the constant stimulus of social media bombarding us with bodacious lifts in 60 second clips without any of the back story of how that lifter trained up to that level. Trust me people, a clip of Larry Wheels smashing 225 lbs incline dumbell benches or the latest Animal cage video from the Arnold never ceases to fire me up, but you must control the urge not to follow your program.

The Harvard folks go on to say that one of the hallmarks of self regulation is the ability of an individual to be open to change. Sounds kind of counter intuitive to believing in your program, but it means that if something did not work for you after you gave it a fair chance, find something else that will work for you. This is the conjugate method at work everyone. As Louie Simmons has famously stated when it comes to training, "everything works but nothing works forever." What got you to a 315 squat will not get you to 405. You must assess, plan and apply new training concepts accordingly to move up the strength ladder.

Motivation is pretty self explanatory to anyone reading this site but let us read for a moment what some Harvard Business experts say about the definition of motivation. "A propensity to pursue goals with energy and persistence." Yes that. Those smart people from Cambridge no doubt have you nodding your head in agreement as that is an awesome definition of what makes a human successful at physical culture. You need goals, both micro and macro, then you need to go after those goals like they tried to steal your significant other-with a vengeance. Optimism even in the face of failure is a hallmark behavioral trait of a motivated person. It takes a somewhat romanticized view of the importance of training to your life to push through at times when your progress has stalled, work and/or school is demanding and general life circumstances seem to be creating frequent roadblocks. A motivated person can achieve amazing results by correctly noting that obstacles are things we encounter when we take our eyes off our goals.

Empathy is the next quality of emotional intelligence that is key to a person reaching the pinnacle of their physical capacity. I state the importance of empathy from experience because the strongest I ever got was when I had serious, dedicated training partners to work out with. Training partners push you at times because no one can be "on" all the time. Training partners allow you to push the heaviest weights possible because they provide a measure of safety when they spot each other when a lifter is pushing her or his limits. Behind 99% of the strongest beings I have met their was a fantastic group of training partners. What do training partners and empathy have to do,with each other? According to Harvard, empathy is "expertise in building and retaining talent." A true strength athlete will find the strongest people to train with as well as grow potential strength athletes along with the meat eater crew they wreck the gym with. As Louie Simmons says, a Ronin is a person who could be a

Samurai but does not pass along the skills he has learned. Don't be a Ronin.

The sport Powerlifting has a long history of older lifters who mentored young kids to become great lifters. I did it with Josh Bryant, Gary Frank used to train with many young football players, and 9 time World Champion Larry Pacifico used to hire potential studs to work in his health spa chains who became world champs such as Joe Ladnier

The final characteristic of an emotionally intelligent individual is someone who possess social skill, which is defined as the ability to find common ground and build rapport. This could be as easy as not tossing a curler from the squat rack if you are in a commercial gym setting but I interpret it to mean train with others regardless if everyone has different goals at the time. The key is that the individuals all have serious personal goals. In my garage gym, I train with two scholarship college football players, Jiu Jitsu fighters, baseball players and a literal rocket scientist who wants to be in the best shape of his life for his wedding. I am the only person whose sole focus is Powerlifting, yet we all thrive because it is like our own private fight club versus the weights. Build a team to help each other with your training and you will never regret it.

Be attuned to your increased emotional intelligence my fellow iron slingers and just ignore anyone who makes the serious mistake of thinking you are all brawn and no brains. That is like thinking that an hour or two of reality television viewing compares to a personal record of any sort. Crazy thought isn't that my fellow iron intellects?

Why did I?

Mike Martin is one of the best training partners and even better friend I have ever had. We live similar life styles but he is twice the man I will ever be. Both Mike and I have followed the Westside Barbell Conjugate Method for the past quarter century. Like many who have followed this method, neither of us, although invited, have never actually trained at Westside Barbell in Columbus. Mike and I will connect with each other through texts or calls and we will often repeat that famous line that Louie Simmons attributes his comeback to the platform

that was uttered to him by Powerlifting god Jesse Kellum, "Why don't you?"

2018 marked my 50th year on this planet as well as my 33rd of entering a Powerlifting or Strongman competition. You learn a few things during a third of a century as a competitive strength athlete. 2018 also marked the 4th year since I pulled an official deadlift of 600 lbs. That is right folks, I first pulled 600 in 1988 but 30 years later I had allowed an entire high school career pass without hauling 6 plates and change. My latest pectoral tendon injury in 2015 resulted in me trying to switch to the hook grip, ala Brad

Gillingham, in an effort to increase my deadlift but not stress my latest upper body injury.

I began working my deadlift hard with the hook grip, but in February 2016, I pulled a set of deadlifts with over 500 lbs and something popped in my left scapula area causing me pain for months as well as numbness in my pinkie and ring finger on my left hand. In addition the long head of my tricep on the left lost its normal tone and now felt mushy. I did a meet a few months later. Why did I? Because the two young lifters I was training at the time, Tavian and Sean were signed up for it already. I stick to my commitments people. Trust me, although I pulled a 573 for a USAPL state record, it was embarrassing to not bench body weight because I could not fire my left tricep. We all know Josh is a bench legend, but in 2000 I was able to beat Josh at the USPF National Bench Championships-the only time my old ass beat my amazing, then teenage training partner.

I trained in 2017 but made minimal improvements. No Dr or therapist in Tucson could helpbut I kept scratching as Chuck Voghelpohl is alleged to have said to Louie. Why did I? I have three kids who compete in football, Jiu Jitsu, volleyball and lift as well. I also had loyal training partners, Tavian and Sean who were entering their senior year of High School football. Both these young men set multiple Arizona State USAPL records and earned college football scholarships.

Tavian and Sean went away to college and I selfishly lost myself in my son's senior year of high school football. Why did I? If I have to explain to you how you can immerse yourself in your kids sports/activities/life-just stop reading now. This is not for you. Friday's took on a whole new life as I would make sure nothing got in the way of my son's varsity football games. My son is by no means a five star recruit, he was third string at best- but he earned the right to carry the football as a running back on a team that won their division in Southern Arizona.

Sunday morning would roll around and I would realize Lou's football career would soon end, so I would train in my garage and deadlift. I often trained with my youngest son Max, who really took to lifting this year. I was not able to train with any other competitors as my focus is on what works best for my family's schedule-period. I follow the well run USAPL Arizona website and I saw a contest announced for December 9th in Tucson. I entered. Why did I? As Louie Simmons says, compete locally often in order to grow the sport or possibly meet new training partners. There was more to it than that though as I let my mind open as to something that is always there, but comes around during the holiday season.

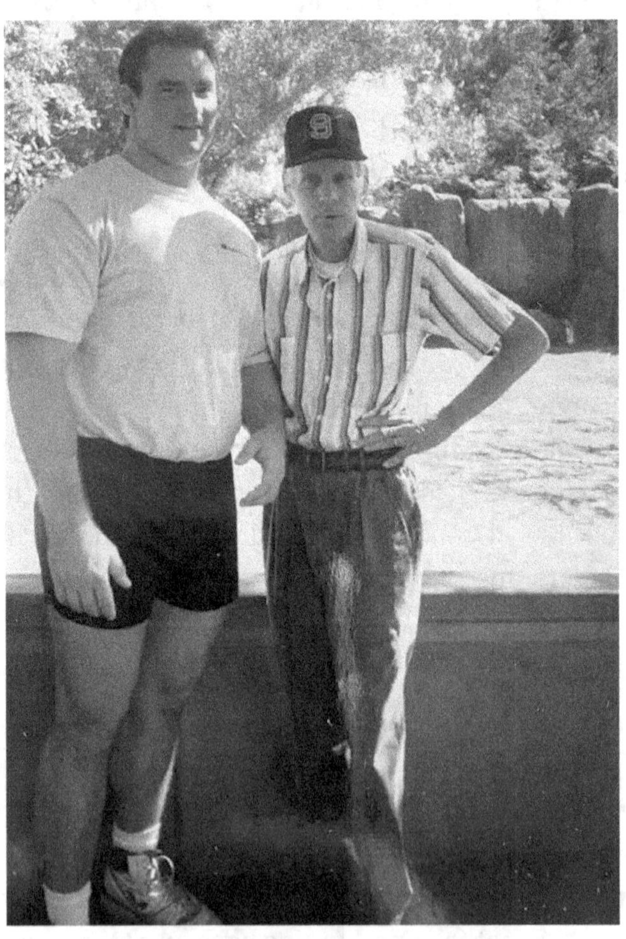

My father died of medical malpractice on Christmas Eve 1998. Ironically my dad suffered from Kyphosis or hunchback and suffered greatly following surgery to correct his back. Sadly, after an operation, my father received dirty blood during a transfusion and the resulting hepatitis killed him. Yes, I am still mad about it today. With the twenty year anniversary of my father's death playing in my mind, I decided to take my seething anger out on a bar. But first I needed to plan my attack as I had not pulled a 600lb deadlift in over 1300 days.

After much reflection, I settled on a program beginning in September where I would pull heavy one week and somewhat lighter the following week. All summer I had tried to copy Brad Gillingham with heavy rack singles as my primary deadlift max effort work. Strike two for me being a distant Gillingham as rack pulls gave me my first case of sciatica. Thankfully

Donnie Thompson's lower back protocol (hanging upside down by the now illegal monster band) as well as John Kuc's leg raise for reps every day rid me of sciatica. Instead of Big Brad, I deduced I would copy 1000lb deadlifted Martin Licis, whose Instagram posts indicated he trained the deadlift in RDL form, squeezing the bar off the floor with less leg drive and saving his biggest pulls for within 8 weeks of a contest. Licis, like Gillingham, advocates RDLs raw to build their posterior chain. The only other twist I added this year was focusing on the negative during a deadlift to give me more muscle building tension-thank you Chad Coy.

My deadlift workouts went as such (Only top set listed/only one "money shot" set doneremember, I am 50 now):

9/2: Safety bar squat to a 12" box with a belt 405x2 reps; deadlift Licis style 412 X 5 reps no belt but straps-pause each rep at the ankle with a 3 second negative each rep.

 9/8: Competition deadlift grip (the old over and under) with a belt, 498 X 5 reps.

9/15: Squat with 14" cambered bar 403X2, Reverse band with blue band (strong) 66" from floor-deadlift with competition grip 623lbs.

9/23: Zercher squat 388lbs X 1 with deadlift stance; Licis style no belt but straps with 440 X 5.

9/30: Safety Bar Squat to 12" box with 415 X 2, reverse band in green (medium bands) 66" off floor up to 610 competition grip deadlift with belt.

10/7: Deadlift raw with competition grip: 450 bar weight plus 40lbs in chains X 3, 450 bar weight plus 68 total in chains x 3 reps for 2 sets. I did the three work sets above in 15 minutes. I try to do multiple work set days within the same time it takes to run a flight of lifts at a meet.

10/14: Competition grip deadlift from floor with belt: 450 X 3, 525 X 3.

10/21: Ironminds Apollon's Axl bar zercher with deadlift stance, work up to 265lbs for 3 wearing a light belt (The old Safe Company belt from Minnesota); Deadlift with competition grip: 360 bar weight with 108 total in chains X 3 reps, 410 bar weight plus 108 in chains X 3 reps- sets. Three deadlift work sets done in 17 minutes.

At this point, with 6 weeks to go, I switched my deadlift day to midweek because I like to pull my last deadlift ten days before a meet. I also begin to note the rate of perceived effort (RPE) a set takes.

10/25: Competition grip deadlift with belt: 470 X 3 (RPE 7), 540 X 3.

10/29: Squat with 14" cambered bar 443 X 2 reps with belt. Bent Over Rows with Safe belt and raw grip: 207lbs 4 sets of 5 reps

10/31: Competition grip deadlifts raw: 407 bar weight plus 108 total in chains X 5 reps, 427 bar weight plus 108 in chains X 4 reps, 457 bar weight plus 108 in chains X 3 reps, 467 bar weight plus 108 in chains X 2 reps. I did the four work sets in 20 minutes. That is a Jon Cole workout. I then proceeded to pig out that night as my wife, son and his girlfriend ate as much candy as we handed out. What a blubbergut I was.

11/3: Safety bar squat to a 12" box with 352lbs bar weight and tight blue bands for a double

(About the time a grinding deadlift would take)

11/7: Competition grip deadlift with power belt: 556lbs for 3 reps (RPE 9). (Heaviest workout of the entire cycle)

11/11: Deload workout in the squat with Safety squat bar and green bands for two sets of triples paused on a 12" box. Snatch grip bent over rows with a safe belt and no straps up to 278lbs for two triples.

11/15: Competition grip deadlift with 450 lbs bar weight plus 108 in chains X 1 no belt. Add Safe belt: 500lbs bar weight plus 108 in chains X 1 rep (RPE 9), 520 bar weight plus 108 in chains X 1 rep (RPE 10).

11/18: Squat with Westside Bow Bar up to 398 lbs to a hassock on 1" 45 lb plate. Used Safe belt and took deadlift stance. All squatting during this training cycle was done with a deadlift stance to build leg drive off the floor. Watch a YouTube video of Eddie Hall squatting some time.

11/22: Thanksgiving morning with Max, Bow bar squat to a hassock on a 1"45 lb plate up to 431 lbs with power belt and knees wrapped; being peaking cycle for deadlift meet with Prilipen's chart figures for Dynamic Effort deadlifts: 500lbs bar weight for 8 singles in 14 minutes wearing a Safe belt and using my competition grip.

11/25: Bent over rows with Safe belt and straps: 228 X 3, 248 X 3 X 2 sets, 268 X 3 reps.

Safety bar deadlift stance good mornings with 135 lbs X 10 reps raw, leg raises X 40 reps

11/29: Dynamic deadlift workout, competition grip and power belt: 517 lbs for 6 singles in 9 minutes. Felt awesome. Recovering and ready to pull big soon.

12/2: Safety bar squat inside power rack to hassock on a 45 lb plate with deadlift stance up to 375lbs for 1 pause rep with power belt; add monster mini bands to the bar overhead to deload the weight in the bottom- 465 lb bar weight x 1 rep. Dimmel deadlifts with straps and no belt: 138lbs X 20 sets of 2 reps done quick to flush back out, decline bench abs with 10lb plate behind head.

12/7: Friday. On a cold, rainy day in Tucson, I attended the funeral of Deputy United States Marshal Chase White who was slain in the line of duty. These type of events are sobering and put life in perspective for me.

12/8: Saturday. I had to buy a new car because one of our cars was totaled on 11/26. No one was hurt. Just my wallet.

12/9: Meet day. Max and I drove over in my old Hemi Charger. The meet site was not well marked but we found it. I weighed in at 126 kilos, or Superheavyweight in the USPAL. I did warms ups of 460 and 515. I opened at 551 then took my goal weight of 600lbs. It was pretty easy and I was super focused for lift-period. I thought about my dad and my Max who was there with me. My last thought before I tightened my belt was that I hope all my kids love something in their life as much as I love lifting weights. Something 100% objective that can never be disputed and will always mean something to those who "get it." I love Henry Rollins wisdom and 200lbs will always be 200 lbs....but so will 600-it is just 3 times better.

I had some close friends at the meet as well, Ray Robey (somehow two alpha males became friends after age 40-like Bigfoot riding the Loch Ness Monster-it can happen!), his son Tavian back from school, and the Barrega Family- who let me train their athletes. My friend and new training partner Mike Alperstein came to support me. Thank you for coming folks.

As for the other type of training I did during the fall of 2018, all of my pressing was incline pressing as my left shoulder inflamed greatly from flat pressing with my football players as they got ready for their season. Lots of miles in them there pecs. I was able to strictly incline bench more weight than I benched in my last full meet in 2016. In addition to focusing on my incline press, I did a great deal of upper body pulling exercises ala Bruce Wilhelm and Bill Starr- with a snatch grip. I have never worked any snatch grip pulls in my lifting career so there were new strength gains to be mined and I was able to strengthen that weak scapula area I strained in 2016. Like the immortal Jon Cole would train very heavy upright rows with 405 then he would enter an Olympic lifting meet and beat everyone but Olympian Kenny Patera.

A few of my peers saw the 600 lb lift and asked....why didn't you go for more? Well Why Did I pass my third attempt? I passed my third because I wanted to save some energy for my family over the holidays. I also passed the attempt so that I could smash some weights a few weeks later on the 20th anniversary of my father's passing. Training is my anchor and I exist to do it.

Since you frequent this site you know Josh has benched more than 620 raw, and many of his clients pull over 800 lbs. My pull is no big deal - to you. I am just an ally and friend of Josh's who became the first USAPL 50 year old in Arizona to pull 600lbs. So now I ask you about your goal, Why don't you?

Powerlifting and strength sports – it is all in your mind!

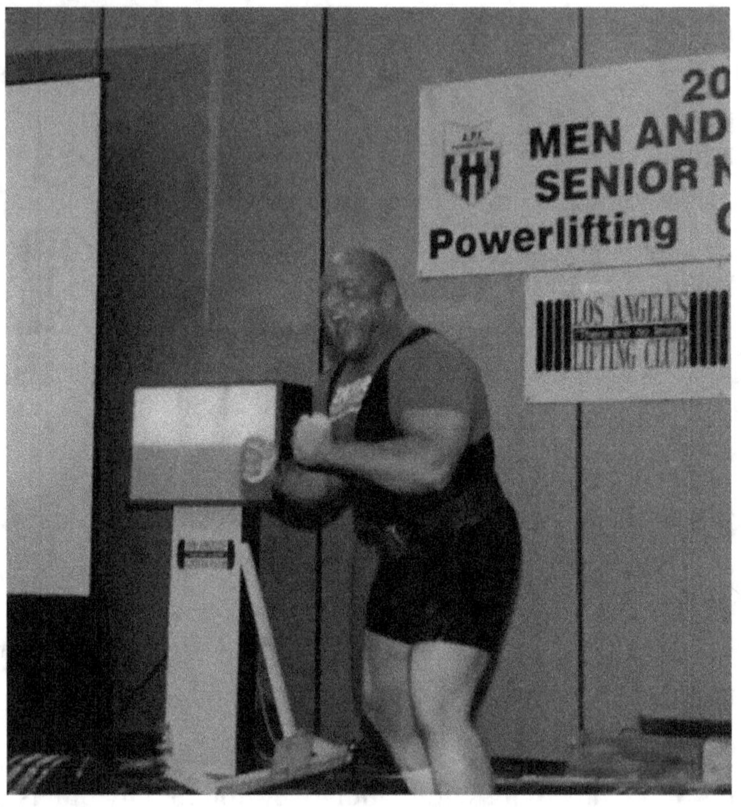

There is a famous clip of Arnold Schwarzenegger talking about how all success in serious strength training all starts in the mind. As a lifter lucky enough to have started out with numerous news stand publications which catered to serious bodybuilders and powerlifters. Numerous bodybuilding magazines, specifically Flex and Muscle and Fitness had articles by Peter Siegel, who was the premiere peak performance hypnotherapist in the U.S., as well as monthly articles by Judd Biasiotto in Powerlifting USA. Dr. Judd was famous for squatting 600 at 132lbs and shared the sports psychology he used for elite lifting in Powerlifting USA. I became very proficient with visualization while in my late teens because the strength publications constantly reminded their readers of the importance of mental training.

In college I read everything I could find about Bill Kazmaier. His training booklets had a handwritten print of his trademark phrase: ***"Conceive, believe, achieve."*** When he was interviewed during the 1982 World Strongest Man Contest, Kaz told the television audience that he was sure he was the strongest man who had ever lived. Confidence has always been a Kazmaier strong point- and he has elaborated many times in interviews that you can find on YouTube, about his belief in visualization. Kaz described during a SWISS Conference Speech that he envisioned that his arms were hydraulic pistons when he bench pressed-this mind and muscle connection led to a half dozen all time world bench press records in the early 1980s.

As I have been a competitive strength athlete for over 35 years, I am aware that many people experience anxiety over performing their sport or from life in general. I myself had a high degree of anxiety when I began junior high school and had to traverse the city of Boston to get to school through the melting pot that is the ethnically and socially diverse city. I got beat up more than a few times while I was 12 and 13, but I soon discovered lifting weights and proper eating. Coupled with joining the football team and falling in love with training- my anxiety was gone by my sophomore year and I loved high school, as well as college. To be quite honest, I had huge success as a teenage powerlifter and I never felt anxiety with my sport or in my life. I know many people are not so fortunate and I also know that anxiety can return in your life- as it did in mine once my children became teenagers. My three children had various issues growing up and I did feel very anxious while I navigated parenting three teenagers while working full time.

What I did, at any time I felt anxiety, was to make sure I trained. Every house I have owned has had a garage gym. My family could always see me train- fit around my work and family responsibilities.

At times all my kids trained with me and I was able to introduce them to what was my anchor in life- training. I would explain to them that when there were issues you could not work on, it was best not to worry about those issues. As for me, I have never had such clarity as I do while the endorphins of a strength training session were coursing through my veins. I also would tell them that mental health is extremely important and that it begins with you controlling your body through training. I modeled and talked about stress management, positive action, consistency, discipline and dedication. I had entered contests every year since 1986, but in 2015 and 2019, I entered no contests because I had family issues and work responsibilities that were far more important than entering any contest- but I still trained as best I could.

I have a vast library regarding strength training and I would study those publications that stressed the mental aspect of strength training and stress management. John McCallum's Keys to Progress, Bill Starr, Marty Gallagher's the Purposeful Primitive, and Brooks Kubik's Dinosaur Training are so classic, go to resources that always give me perspective.

More recently Josh Bryant, unequivocally the most successful strength athlete to become a world class coach, has written extensively in many of his Jailhouse Strong books, articles and blog entries on Joshstrength about the importance of mental training. Josh and I learned from each other how to train our minds to be like steel traps, impervious to pain, injuries, training in extreme climates as well as training following extensive travel. Josh was a close personal friend of the late, great Fred Hatfield, PHD and known as Dr. Squat following his 1014 squat at age 46 and only 257 lbs. Dr. Squat wrote often about the mental health one needs to cultivate and maintain to optimize one's strength and performance.

It is 2021 and now there must be dozens of apps which help athletes with their mental training process. I have not explored these tools as I have mastered the art of visualization for me. I highly recommend you invest the time in training your mind even more often than you train your body.

Seven things I re-learned

1.   Everybody Wants Some, the title of this quintessential 80s rock song from Van Halen brings back pleasant memories of driving too fast and the movie Better Off Dead, a great snapshot of teenage angst. The song also contains the line...”Yeah that’s it, a little more to the right...”. David Lee Roth crooned that line to paint the picture of woman who was the epitome of sensuality, while a male enjoyed the view. I am here to tell you fellow ironslingers that an inch or so can make a huge difference in the gym.

This past year, I read an article by Louie Simmons that the great Doug Heath cured his shoulder ailment by placing a ten pound plate under either the head of his flat bench or under the feet of the bench, creating either the smallest incline or decline. I did this for 2 months and my shoulder inflammation disappeared. I should have remembered that an inch or so can make a big difference.

2.   Regarding Louie Simmons, this year I saw the documentary Westside bs the World. If you look closely at the ten minute mark you will see my arm putting up the great Art Labare’s squat suit strap at the inaugural WPO meet in Daytona Beach, circa 2000. I was heavily influenced by Louie and the Westside content that he created in the 1990s, specifically his articles and video tapes. I recently found an entire box of these old articles and they are filled with training gold. In my opinion the conjugate principles that these articles contain are a great way for a raw lifter such as myself to train. If you can find these materials, I highly suggest you study them for very useful information on training percentages, volume, and unique exercises to implement. One gem Louie wrote in an article from that era was “At Westside we do a lot of a few things.”

3.   Rack work is great for my squat and pressing exercises. I have come back from numerous surgical repairs of my pectoral

tendons as well as a tricep reattachment. I did this by utilizing power rack training as described by Josh with the dead bench, Anthony Ditillo, and Brad Gillingham. What I regret doing is stopping rack lockouts and partial range of motion pressing once I got back to my pre-surgery level of strength. When you press from a rack position it is pure concentric exercise with no eccentric stress. I really enjoy training with partial overload work and from a dead stop position. Eric Fiorillo of the Podcast Motivation and Muscle recently described power rack training as proving the trainee with infinite opportunities to progress. My sentiment exactly!

4.   I enjoy listening to podcasts and there are many to chose from in you seek great training information. The great John Welbourn recently stated on his podcast that most trainees fail to improve because they ignore the three pillars of training which are to implement Hatfield's compensatory acceleration, incorporate isometric work to increase stability, and utilize the medicine ball plyometric exercises recommended by Ben Johnson's strength coach Charlie Francis. I read and study any content from Hatfield and you should too. No man on earth ever got more out of his body than Dr Squat.

5.   The book Dinosaur Training which was published in 1996 is a great book which needs to be read by every garage gorilla, cellar dweller, raw power lifter and drug free trainee. I have seen some of Mr Kubic's more recent work but I much prefer the classic Dinosaur book which will soon be a quarter of a century old. Rack work, thick bars, sandbags, finishing moves, mindset training, grip work, and attitude are what you will re-learn if you have not visited this book in too long.

6.   Stiff leg deadlifts should always be done. I am writing this article on the 19 year anniversary of George Brink's epic 804 lb deadlift at the USPF Nationals in Burbank at age 51! George had a back of steel and a torso like a Grizzly bear. He would do extensive

cycles of stiff leg deadlifts off blocks for 5 sets of 10 reps. George was a good inch taller than me at over 6'3" and his back was as broad as an axe handle or two. I leave a slight bend in my knee and I squeeze the weight off the floor with my posterior chain. I slow the eccentric down to between 3 to 5 seconds to build as much muscle as possible. Wear straps and use a front grip so the emphasis is on building your erectors and nothing else.

7.   Life is fleeting and should be enjoyed while you try your best to leave a legacy of sharing your passions with others. When I heard that the world had lost Franco Columbo, I was shocked that he could die. There is a video online from a few years ago of Arnold describing how Franco's muscle tissue was unlike anything Arnold had ever seen on another human. He was, pound for pound, one of the strongest men to ever grace the earth. By all accounts he was also one of the most beloved members of the Golden Era bodybuilders.

Franco died doing what he must have loved doing-swimming off the coast of Sicily this summer. What a fitting way for him to pass as only the power of the ocean could overcome his physical being.

Weight Gain For MEN – A Serious Matter

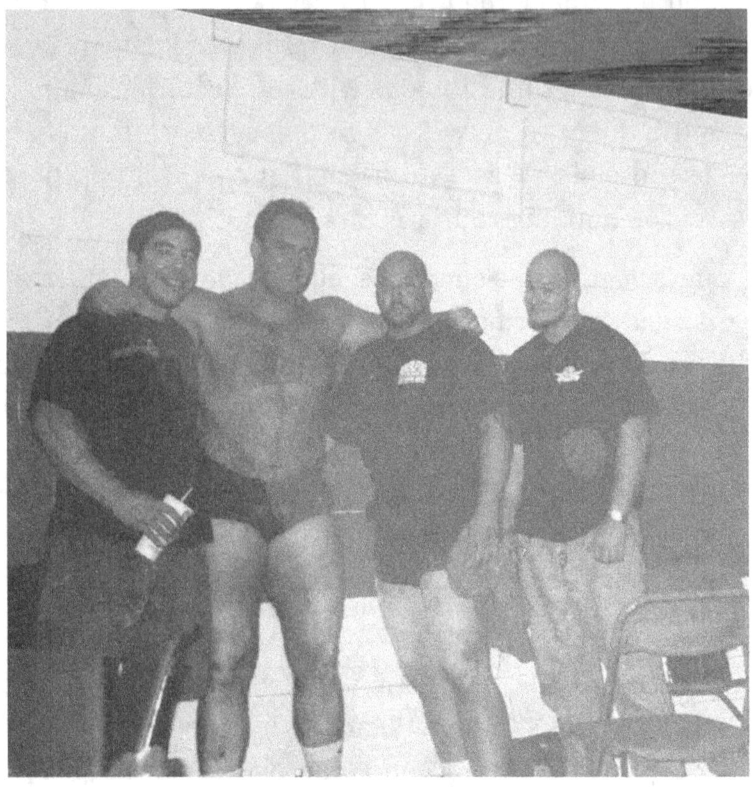

I was born premature and weighed only 4lbs and 6 ounces. As I was born to a Catholic family, I was given my last rites and named Joseph in the event I died, which I did not. Once I stuck around I was renamed Paul. I had a normal healthy childhood, loving playing baseball, swimming, building forts and always with lots of friends and activities. I loved to climb trees and I can recall running around day in the summer until my legs would ache when I came home to eat and sleep once it was dark. I ate very well growing up with my mother feeding us well and my grandmother living in the same building as us so two of every meal swas the norm for me and I entered junior high school as a chubby kid.

I loved to eat healthy food as well as junk food. I was a paperboy and made my own money that I spent on baseball cards and snacks at the local convenience stores. Candy, slushes, and soda pop was consumed in between meals.

Once in high school, after having been beat up and jumped more than I cared for commuting by busses and trains throughout Boston, I decided to build myself up by lifting weights and eating better. I had no one to teach me how to lift the first year I did, but I recall the 110lb cement filled weight set I received from my parents in 1982 came with a booklet to follow.

I began to lift weights with my high school football teammates and became a starter on the varsity team at 6'2" and 215lbs. I loved to eat while I was in high school and worked part time jobs that made it possible to eat lots. I worked for Burger King for 4 months and ate Whoppers, then I worked at a nursing home in the kitchen where food was plentiful, followed by a stint with a local pizza parlor at which I ate a pizza every day I worked, covered with extra cheese, gyro meat as well as meatballs and sausages. I walked a lot in high school as my parents wouldn't let me buy a car until I graduated.

I began powerlifting in earnest as soon as my high school football career ended and by then I began reading strength and bodybuilding magazines like Powerlifting USA, Ironman, Muscle and Fitness, Musclemag International, Muscular Development, Flex, MuscleTraining Illustrated, and some books as well.

I realized the importance that nutrition played in building muscle to lift heavier weights. I also began to use supplemental protein such as Weiders Muscle Builder and GNC's store brand. Most of my diet was food.

In college, with more money and fully obsessed with getting as strong as I could get, I began to eat more food and supplements. I flew down to compete in a huge competition in Maryland and came in 2nd to a beast named Shawn Colbeth who became a Collegiate National Champion and his ass kicking of me opened my eyes to how intense a person could be on the platform. I was 19 and squatted 515 benched 315 and deadlifted 560 in the 242 lb class.

Shawn did a 600lb and deadlifted 600, benching 480. We wore single ply gear and were drug tested as this contest was sanctioned by the American Drug Free Powerlifting Association (ADFPA), which today is the USAPL, the U.S's IPF affiliate.

The ass kicking did not deter me at all, rather it spurred me on to train as hard as I could. I followed Fred Hatfields Programs from Muscle And Fitness as well as did Dr Ken Leistner's workouts. I once squatted 315 for 20 reps and then passed out on the toilet for about 30 minutes afterwards. I did meets in the 242 and 275lb class in 1988 and 1989. In 1988 I began working for GNC as a sales associate while in college. I sold tons of supplements and was allowed to sample everything GNC sold.

I worked for GNC for over two years. I would work alone so I could not leave to eat in the mall I worked at so I became heavily involved in eating supplements. It was not uncommon for me to eat 50 amino acid capsules or tablets along with the same amount of desiccated liver tablets in the same 4 hour shift. I often worked 5 to 9 pm close. There were no ready to drink protein supplements at that time, but I would bring a quart of milk with me to the job and we had single serving packets of protein powder to mix in. Protein powder then was primarily calcium caseinate.

Some of the brands I hammered then were Universal, Unipro, Hot Stuff, Twinlab,

MegaPro,and at times GNC's competitor Nature Food Center's store brand. I ate everything I could get my hands on and I just got stronger, with my powerlifting total going up from 1250 at 18 to 1600 at 21 and 235lbs. What I did not gain was a great amount of bodyweight in those 3 years. What was missing was food!

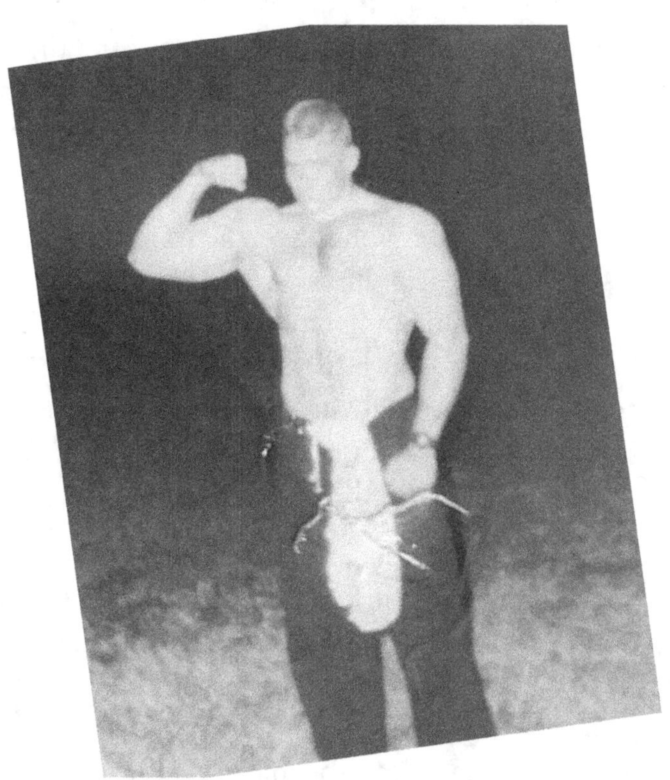

I graduated college and moved to Southern California to begin my career. I had to meet certain physical standards to include a mile and a half in a fast time so I maintained a weight of 220. In 1993, I was established in my career and determined to pursue my powerlifting goals. I also began Westside Barbell style training, which was higher volume an intense pace that put me in great shape but I couldn't get past 262lbs after a year.

Enter the food in 1995. After finishing 2nd in the 275 lb class in the 1995 USPF California States with lifts of 661 413 705 at 262lbs, I settled down personally and got married. My lifting goals were now around getting as large and strong as possible- no longer was my focus just on strength, I wanted to get as muscular and big as possible.

I had a fantastic training crew and a supportive wife who cooked for me and gave me all the sex I wanted. No other iron game writer other than Bill Starr ever wrote about sex and the barbell, but I will say it- I had lots of sex since I was 16 and even more after I got married. Nothing made me grow like great training, real food and sex before bed or after a great workout.

Between 1995 and 1998 my body weight went from 262 to 325, with my lifts going to official lifts of 771 480 744. The keys were this: Sunday was food shopping day and a day off the gym. Often times I would get up and eat a breakfast at home like eggs, milk, pancakes, toast, and some fruit. Sex and then back to bed again for a few hours. My wife and I would then go to brunch, there was a place in So Cal called Charley Browns that had a great brunch.

I can eat insane amounts of food, if I keep changing the type of food. Prime rib, lobster, shrimp, Turkey, potatoes,rice, you get the idea. This restaurant served NFL brunch so while an NFL game played, my goal was to eat at least one huge plate of food (1000 calories) for every quarter of the game. At home after brunch either more sex and a nap- in the summer in my pool or inside during the fall. When it got dark we would go to the supermarket and spend our 300 dollars for the week for the two of us. My wife never weighed more than 110lbs until she got pregnant but she is a great cook and ate very well too.

My training spilt to gain that weight was Monday was speed bench, Tuesday was speed squat, Thursday was max effort bench and Saturday morning was max effort lower body lifts- primarily focused on the deadlift.

After Saturday's training we would go to Rocky Cola Cafe in Uptown Whittier to eat off both the regular menu and the health food menu. I would eat egg white enhanced French toast, a peanut milkshake made with Metrx, then I would eat a Buffalo meat burrito and wash it down with an apple pie Metrx shake.

I would drive home and grab the wife for sex after a shower then a nap in my pool or while watching college football. Nighttime involved a dinner out, often times at Black Angus Steak house or at

Claim Jumper- getting a dinner called the Ore Cart which had over 5,000 calories of meat and sides of stuffed baked potatoes. Desert was often Golden spoon Frozen Yogurt, as I was a member of the quart club- buy 9 and the tenth was free.

During the week day, I had to work but I would eat in accordance to my goal. **Breakfast** was always a steak, eggs, orange juice, milk, and bagels with peanut butter. I would always have food with me at work. I love nuts, peanuts, almonds, and **Arnold's favorite- cashews**. I would often drink milk- up to a gallon per day on days not in the gym, not as much as gym days as I did not want to feel lactose sluggish.

I drove 42 miles,one way to work, so I knew all the places to eat along the way if I got hungry. I would eat El Pollo Loco Chicken, Rubios, Jamba Juice, Togo's, and other local restaurants. I ate almost zero fast food.

I had a few local restaurants that really helped me out. La Salsa at the Glendale Galleria had a sweet lady named Maria would would make a burrito as big as my 17" forearm loaded with steak, rice, and cheese. Chuys in Glendale offered a lunch buffet that was amazing. All you could eat tri tip roast and mesquite grilled chicken for 9.99 per day! Host Ted and server Katarina became fast friends and appreciated how strong and big I got.

At the time there was a famous picture of Professional Body Builder Lee Priest eating KFC to bulk up. I would do the same occasionally, but I would throw away the covering as to digest all that fried shit would have slowed me down.

Every 12 weeks I would go to Lindberg Nutrition at the Del Amo Fashion Center in Torrance with my wife. I would buy creatine, glutamine, amino acids, whey protein- Designer Whey, desiccated liver, and ultimate orange for energy. I would take 20 grams of creatine, glutamine, BCAAs, prior to and half way through each workout. After my three weekday workouts, my wife would have dinner for me when I got home and before bed I would have a pound of yogurt with whey protein mixed in it with some ovaltine. I slept for about 7 hours per week night and more on the weekend with naps whenever I wanted as I had no kids then.

I had an amazing physician who supported my goals and monitored all my blood work, blood pressure, cholesterol, and key indicators such as liver enzymes and kidney function. If I had not been healthy, I would never have gotten as large and strong as I did. When I began competitive strongman in 2001, I ceased trying to gain weight and I began losing body fat I had gained when I gained 60lbs in 3 years. That was over twenty years ago and I am as healthy as ever at 53. I hope you understand that I was able to gain weight and strength for one reason: I loved the process and I would do it all again.

How I DEFEATED Mike O'Hearn at Powerlifting Competition

The 1995 USPF State Powerlifting Championships were held on April 22, 1995, at the El Toro Marine Air Corp Station. Twenty five years later, I found the VHS copy of the meet that was filmed, edited and sold by Guy Adams. The meet was promoted by Vic Elliot, who was an outstanding lifter himself. The competition was held in the basketball gymnasium while the warm up area was the adjacent weight room. The contest was important to me because I had been following the **Westside Barbell training protocol** as best I could by having never been to Westside. I say trying to follow it because as the lifters from Westside and founder Louie Simmons himself say, if you have never trained at Westside than you are not training Westside. In the mid 90s, Louie's video tapes, writings, and recommended reading list of Russian authors were my sources of inspiration.

I had received the 3 original Westside tapes for Christmas of 1993 and began applying the ideas with a shit ton of balls out effort, mostly training alone in a office space at night after work, once everyone had left for the work day. I had a 1600 lb total when I started Westside style and in one year I officially totaled 1717 at the 1994 USPF Vandenberg Air Force Bass Open in the 275 lb class. Soon after that, I relocated to the North Orange County area and began training at a real gym, Uptown Gym in Whittier that had an existing Powerlifting crew.

When I showed up at the gym, the lifters there were split in that two of them (Gary Hogan and Mike Morgan) wanted to train **Westside style like me**, while three of them were vehemently opposed to Westside and said it would not work (Al Morentin, Ray Cosio, and Ron Perkins).

How We Trained For Power

I lead the way with Gary and Mike, using a dynamic effort (DE) day for both squat and bench pressing, as well as a max effort (ME) day for the bench and squat/deadlift as well. Our split called for ME lower on Saturday, ME bench on Thursday, DE bench on Monday, and DE squats on Tuesday. We did no training on our off days, but I trained as hard as I could the 4 days per week that I did hit the gym- balls to the wall and no deloads at that time, just Louie's percentages on DE days and go as heavy as you could til you missed on ME day.

Of all the days, our **Tuesdays** were the worst, with literally ten minutes of terror as we would do all our DE squats sets, 10 or 12 sets of doubles to a 12" box with a medium stance and only a belt. Basically we would do the sets while **AC DC blared Hell's Bells** and **Have a Drink on Me** or **Rage Against the Machine** screeched a Bullet to the Head or Calm like a Bomb. Ten minutes of music, 10 or 12 doubles as hard as we could apply compensatory acceleration to each rep-ala Fred Hatfield whom Louie revered. Chains and bands were not used nor where they known about by myself in 1995.

After DE squats we would do power good mornings to build up our back static strength for a big squat. With 365 to 405 for triples with a belt, I was able to squat 700lbs in competition with ease after training this way for two years. After good mornings we would do cable pull throughs with up to our respective bodyweight for hamstring isolation. I would alternate stance width, from medium to wide, digging my heels into the floor and focusing on my hip extending hamstrings. Uptown Gym has a 400 lb heavy duty cable stack that would allow us to overload and isolate our leg biceps. Side bends for the obliques followed as they hit the side muscles and hip insertions hard while tractioning the lower back for the heavy ME lower back based work to follow 4 days later on **Saturday.**

Tuesday's workouts were completed like every other workout, with conditioning. We would do heavy abdominal work supersetted with either ad hoc reverse hypers or Dimel deadlifts. On days we did lower body work, we would condition with sit up type work on either the floor, a hyper bench or a decline bench. On upper body days, abdominal conditioning was done with leg raises, floor, hanging, or on a ramp to open up that lower back for the posterior chain work to follow in the workout to follow the upper session. The gym did not have a reverse hyper, we cut a leather weight belt so that you could slide 25lb Olympic plates on to the belt and do the movement by setting up on a regular hyper extension bench with your feet able to swing underneath and back behind the body.

Monday's DE bench press day was completed on Monday evening. We followed the typical prescribed 65% for 8 sets of 3 reps on the flat bench with three different grips, two closer than my regular competition grip so that my triceps got extra work. I would wear gear at the 1995 State Championships, but 95% of my training was done raw. Following my bench sets I would do tricep extensions such as Paul Dicks presses and rolling dumbbell extensions. Deltoids were trained with plate raises, Bradford presses, and one arm strict side raises. Lat pull downs or chest supported rows were done for lats and upper back strength. After hammer curls, conditioning was done with Dimel deadlifts for 20 reps or reverse hypers, supersetted with leg raises.

Thursday evening was max effort bench with some of the staple exercises being floor press and board presses. A bench shirt was put on once per month in order to gauge progress. Heavy dumbbell bench presses for reps on the flat bench were done as a supplemental exercise following working up to a heavy single ME rep. I would do lat work following the pressing, focusing on upper back work and not tiring my lower back for **Saturday's** onslaught. As with every workout, conditioning was done to complete the days training with lower back and ab work.

Saturday morning meant no work that day, just an ass kicking lower body workout that would include a ME variation squat such as a parallel bench squat , Zercher squat, kneeling squat, or a close stance, sub-12" hassock squat. Following a ME record squat, we would deadlift conventionally using Prilepin's chart as written in an article by Louie titled so you want to deadlift.

It was a 6 week cycle which called for 15 singles pulled with 65%, 12 singles with 70%, 10 singles with 75%, 8 singles with 80%, and finally 6 singles with 85%. These deadlifts were done with a belt and competition grip only. These pulls were done as furious as the DE squats on Tuesdays. I do recall that I pulled 605lbs for 6 singles in 8 minutes – doing this workout ten days before the meet. I ended up pulling 705 at the meet so doing DE deadlifts on ME squat day worked great.

Leading up to the meet, there was friction in the gym as half the team was not training Westside style. The meet would be the test of whose training system was better- my version of Westside or the old school, progressive overload method the other half of the powerlifters were using. There was also lots of shit talking as to who would lift what. There was mention in the contemporary bodybuilding magazines of some of the Gold's Gym Powerlifters of the day, such as how **Mike O'hearn, Ron Fedkiw, Jon Arenberg, and Kurt Elder** we're preparing for the State Powerlifting meet by hoisting impressive poundages in training.

At the time, bodybuilding magazines were popular and **Flex, Muscular Development, Ironman, and MuscleMag International** had columns that would occasionally mention bodybuilders who practiced the power lifts with respectable weights, often times at Golds Gym Venice Beach. I had read bodybuilding magazines since I began lifting weights in 1984.

Weider's magazines, Ironman, Muscular Development, Strength and Health, and MuscleMag International always had at least one piece of content per issue that would help a burgeoning strength fanatic such as myself. While in college I worked at two GNC stores so I would peruse the pages during the slow times- seeking information on how to get stronger, bigger and more muscular. I do not know when I first saw Mike O'hearn in a magazine, but I am sure it was in 1990 or 1991 while I was selling protein, Hot Stuff, or Cybergenics.

The first time I saw Mike O'hearn in person was when he was working the front door of a nightclub, I believe called Club H20, in Manhattan Beach, California on Friday evening November 19, 1993. How do I remember the date so well?

I was invited to Royce Gracie's victory party for winning the first UFC in Denver the Friday before. My room mate rolled with the Gracies in Jiu Jitsu so I was invited. I congratulated Royce and met the scariest man in the world at the same time- his older brother Rickson (Search him on YouTube). I did not meet Mike but I saw him enjoying being a doorman, flirting with some girls. I was a doorman too so I know the deal. Perks of the job.

1995 California State Powerlifting Championships

It has been a quarter of a century, but I remember many parts of the contest well. I drove down the 40 minutes from my condo with Gary Hogan as it was all business. My fiancé got to the sight later with Gary's wife and sat with all team members wives or girlfriends. I recall warming up, and as was my philosophy, I was there to hit PRs in all three lifts and go as close to 9 for 9 as possible. At a meet I am always just concerned about me- as that is the only person I can control. I have always been a better deadlifter so my goal would be to check the sub totals after the last bench and determine what I would need to pull on my third attempt to place as high as possible.

I took my two scoops of Ultimate Orange and warmed up. I proceeded to **squat 617, 644,** and **661** for 3 successes. Benches were disappointing in that I went **396, 413, and 424** but got reds on the third attempt for a lift I thought was good. I was behind my friend Steve Denison and Mike O'hearn at subtotal.

One thing about the Westside style of training, I was very well conditioned for a powerlifter. I never got tired during a meet once I trained Westside, as the workouts were so much more severe than any contest. The reason for this was because I would train with short rest periods, making the weak muscle fibers fire off before they had recovered. **Weaknesses could not hide.**

To rest 10 or 15 minutes between one squat was very easy and allowed me to rage against the bar. I was able to **deadlift 644, 683, and 705 to beat Mike** and place second to Steve.

How strong is Mike O'Hearn?

Mike's official Powerlifting Numbers that day were **Squat 650lb (295kg), Bench 451lb (204kg) and Deadlift 650lb (295kg).** I out deadlifted both Mike and Steve and hit the last big deadlift of the entire meet as no other heavy division lifter hit all 3 pulls, or even took three attempts. You can hear Ray Cosio encourage me before my last pull. The three members of my team were total converts to the Westside style after that meet.

The aftermath

I met and impressed World Class Powerlifter Art LaBare at this meet as well as his partners Gary Garcia, Rick Purchase, Manny Sanchez, George Pessel, and Brian Meek. Those guys became my new training partners soon after, with only Gary staying by my side. We all went on to lift the greatest weights we ever would lifting out of my garage Yorba Barbell over the next decade after the 95 California States.

I never competed against Mike O'hearn again, although I tried by entering every big California meet in Powerlifting and Strongman until I left the State in 2004.

I have every Powerlifting USA Magazine ever printed, all 420 issues beginning in 1977 and ending sadly in 2012. I have the issue that documents this state meet. My performance that day lead me to being interviewed and appearing on Ned Low's Powerlifter Video Magazine and appearing in PLUSA in Ned's and Dr Ken Leistner's Columns.

Once I achieved success in Powerlifting, I gave back to the sport by writing articles for Powerlifting USA as well as other publications.

Strength Training Motivation In My 50s!

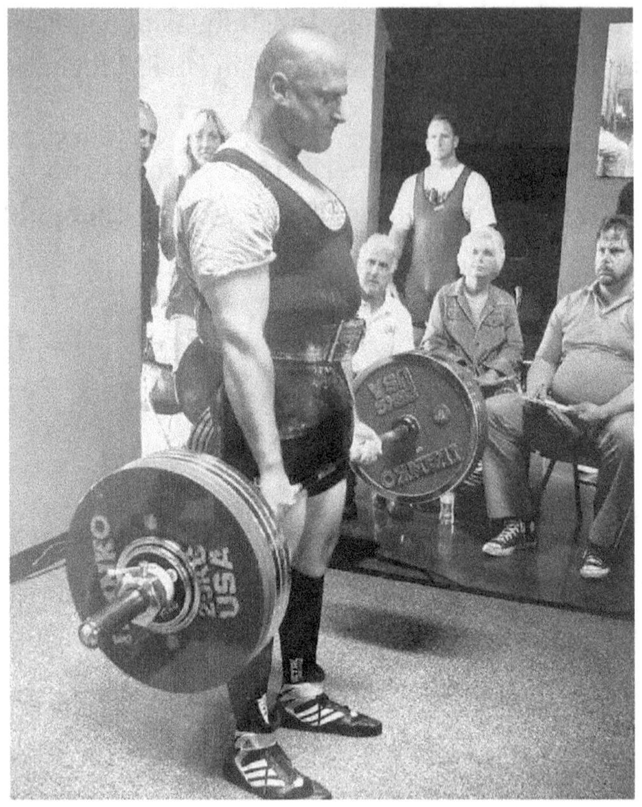

BF with my 628 Deadlift that was an AZ State Record on 7/31/10 at the State Championships

I am a staunch proponent of having a garage or basement gym. I had one as a teenager and then a garage gym was the focus when I bought my first house in California, as well as every house I have bought there after. As the world was forced to stay in their homes during the current pandemic, I decided to venture out and join a commercial gym here in Tucson, Arizona for a variety of reasons. First and foremost, the gym landscape here has changed significantly since I arrived in 2008 – and definitely for the better.

There are now numerous facilities in town which have the proper equipment and members for you to train with for powerlifting, strongman, or bodybuilding but I have found the fit for me to be Beaststrong Powerhouse, with two 24/7, 365 days per year full access facilities, one on each side of town.

I had primarily trained in my garage here and at times it would be over 100 degrees in there. I finally admitted that by the end of a Tucson summer, I was depleted and not making gains due to the extreme heat, humidity, and flying insects associated with a Tucson summer, aka the city's monsoon season. Switching to an air conditioned climate has allowed me to train longer and harder without being so depleted both physically and mentally.

The equipment at my disposal now is far superior to anything I could fit and afford in my two car garage. Reverse hypertension machines, Strongman yokes, various farmers walk implements, sleds, sandbags, kegs, axles, belt squats, bars, bands, chains, wagon wheels, plate loaded rowing machines, Mag lat bars, Smith machines and dumbbells to 155lbs each. The equipment is in excellent shape and spread out, unlike my garage gyms have been. As I have gotten older, I realize the need to stay healthy and build my cardiovascular system. I do not like traditional cardio such as running or treadmill work, but as Louie Simmons, Mike Martin, and the writings of Ken Leistner and John McCallum have taught me- your cardio can be improved by doing supersets or giant sets of assistance exercises for lagging muscle groups with little or no rest between the various exercises.

I recall reading a quote by the immortal Bill Pearl, who turned 90 last October,

"the body does not care how your heart rate increased while training, just that it did."

I look at many of the bodybuilders from the 1970s and 80s who did high volume work and many still look great today- **Arnold, Rory Leidelmeyer, Bill Grant, Dave Draper, and John Hansen.**

Unlike past years, I am able now to spread out and set up equipment and cycle through 4 or 5 exercises such as a chest supported row, a rear deltoid fly, a straight arm pull down then shrugs for high reps. This acceptance of a different training philosophy has given me new goals and muscle mass for my efforts.

Although I did pull a 600 lb deadlift in a USAPL meet to celebrate turning 50, I now enjoy training more than competing. I remember when Jon Cole began training heavy again in his 50s, he told Herb Glossenbrenner that he thrives on training, he needed it's structure. I could not agree more. I still need goals, but training related goals work well for me now as opposed to the constraints of training for a competition, when you have done so for over 35 years.

Dave Shaw always said when his competition career ended he was going to focus on noncompetitive lifts such as the seated military and other lifts he found interesting and still effective for maintaining his muscle mass as he aged. Dave used to come by the Original Orange County Strength Club when I trained there and he was extremely well built and muscular in his 50s.

I love the internet for allowing me to connect with former training partners as well as with great competitors who are still the strongest in the world into their 50s and beyond. A few examples of people whom I connect with through social media for advice are Donny Thompson, Dan Kovacs and Beau Moore. Asa Barnes of Preacher Barbell in Phoenix is a legacy as his father was an all time world record holder and multiple time national champion- and Asa is a fantastic masters level lifter himself today who always provides advice if needed.

For inspiration, David Ricks recently posted a squat video of him repping out with 622lbs at age 62!

As anyone who reads my material knows, I am a huge Jon Cole fan. I posted about Jon on my Instagram recently and a man here in

Arizona commented how many times he would see Jon Cole on a ten speed bike, cruising down University Ave in Tempe after leaving Thorbecke's Gym to go to the gym at Arizona State University to finish his workout. **This got me to train multiple times per day, some training at my house and some training at Beaststrong Powerhouse.** I am making gains, losing fat, regaining strength following some injuries and having fun! As Louie Simmons says, **" training should be fun, heaven or hell is all in your own mind."**

I have heard on Louie's podcast how Westside used to speed bench at a man named Tim Van Horn's house on Sunday morning, then go to a commercial gym to finish their assistance.

The biggest influence on keeping me motivated this year has been the owners of Beaststrong Powerhouse Rafe Teich and his wife. Rafe just won the Overall Men's Bodybuilding Championship at the NPC Europa UBU Expo title in Phoenix in August. He is currently preparing for the North American Championships in his attempt to go professional. His wife, Melissa Teich is an IFBB Professional Bodybuilder who is preparing for the Miss Olympia.

Recent footage on her Instagram page shows her benching 235 for 7 reps and deadlifting over 405 and heavy chains, just a few weeks from the Olympia! Both these individuals inspire me with their positive attitudes, competitive success, dedication to their gyms and their love of the iron. Passion to me is infectious and Beaststrong Powerhouse, from its owners, to its competitors, it's equipment and commitment to personal improvement has been the biggest motivator for me to train hard and ignore the fact I have been training and competing for almost 40 years.

Oldtime- Exercises You Have To Know

Floor Press – Its History and IMPLEMENTATION

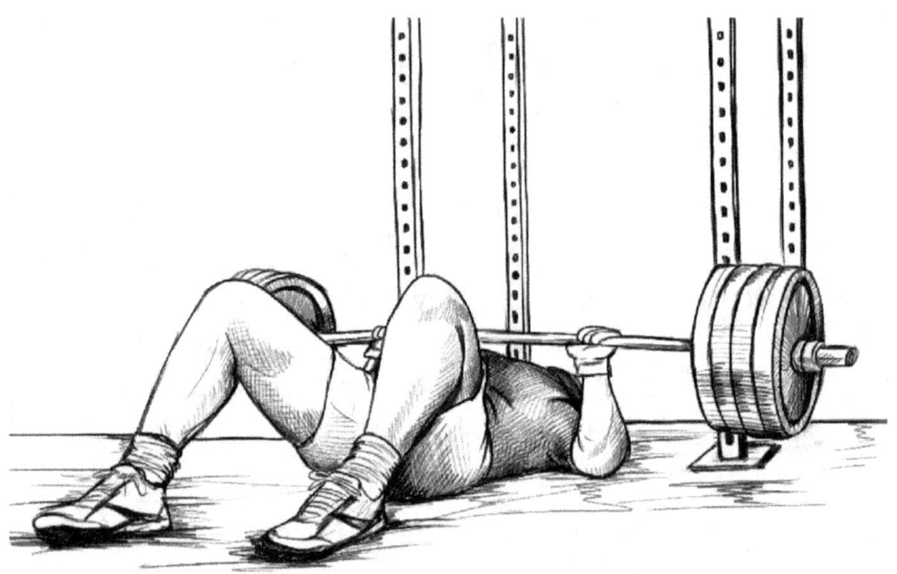

My personal history regarding the floor press began when I read about it in Louie Simmons early 1990s articles. A 1995 article by Louie published in the strength journal Milo, gives credit to Powerlifting legend Jesse Kellum for reminding Louie of how beneficial this exercise is for upper body strength gains.

I have no doubt, that as Charles Poliquin has said, nothing is new in weight training, it has all been done since the turn of the 19th Century. That being said, before commercial bench presses became a common piece of gym equipment in the 1960s, lifters were doing presses on the floor in the early 1900s. Regardless of the origin, floor presses took off after Louie Simmons programmed them in his articles as well as the video tape series he released throughout the 1990s.

Westside Barbell was synonymous with big bench pressers in the 1990s and all of their bench stars were shown in pictures or on video using the floor press to build their prodigious power. Lifters such as Kenny Patterson and George Halbert, who both held all time world records in the bench press wearing a bench press shirt, both could floor press over 600lbs raw. Lifters around the world, myself included, followed suit and did the floor press religiously in their monthly Westside bench template.

Although the floor press was programmed as a max effort exercise that was trained to a maximum single for the workout, lifters soon began to implement the max effort floor press in other manners, such as by adding accommodating resistance with bands, chains or both! The first man to total 3000lbs and bench over 900 while doing it, Donnie Thompson, wrote articles in which he programmed the floor press as a dynamic effort exercise in which he would use 50% of his maximum for 10 sets of triples done as explosively as possible- with or without chains as accommodating resistance.

As Westside evolved during the 2000s, Louie and others such as Ryan Kennelly began writing about doing more and more repetition effort exercises to build muscle mass- with the floor press being a key exercise to program for repetition effort sets.

The floor press can be performed effectively with a lifters competition grip as well as with a close grip for even more tricep emphasis. I know from personal experience, that the floor press was most effective when it was programmed for 5 sets of 5 reps after dynamic effort benches. The reason for this is because the pectorals and anterior deltoids do not fully recover 3 days after a maximum effort pressing workout, but the triceps are fully recovered. The floor press focuses on the triceps due to its limited range of motion- so it is a great exercise to do on the dynamic day which happens 72 hours after the max effort bench day.

I also know from experience that if your shoulders are sore, the floor press makes your shoulders feel great with all of that surface area to press off- as compared with benching on a 12" wide bench. When I competed in strongman and my legs took a beating from all the yoke, drag, farmers walks training- it felt great to get off my feet to build my pressing strength with the floor press. The same can be programmed for athletes like football players and wrestlers. Today, with raw powerlifting far more popular than benching with a shirt, the floor press is even more essential because it is always trained raw. Add the floor press to your workout program and watch your upper body power and development soar.

Dumbbell Pullovers - A foundational movement for mass

Pullover! Now who wants to hear that when they are driving? Not me, but that one time when my wife called it out during our honeymoon in Maui so we could hop in a deserted waterfall that was alright with me. In today's modern strength training athlete's toolbox it appears the traditional dumbbell pullover has been forgotten as a mass maker extraordinaire. Like many lifters who were influenced in the 80s by Arnold Schwarzenegger, I began doing pullovers as soon as I began lifting 35 years ago. I know that doing this base building movement allowed me to build a significantly larger rib cage, wider lats, thicker triceps, and more mobile shoulders. A larger muscle has the potential to be a stronger muscle and that is what eventually happened with me as I began competitive Powerlifting three years after beginning to train. The base I built allowed me to enter strength competitions for the next thirty years.

If you are a younger strength athlete, begin doing pullovers immediately because the soft tissue of your rib cage, serratus muscle, intercostals, and shoulders can be permanently enlarged and strengthened by properly performed pullovers.

Pullovers can be coupled with breathing squats to further harness the natural anabolic power of the squat. A set of squats for 20 reps immediately followed by a set of cross bench pullovers for 10 reps allows the lifter to stretch the rib cage due to the heavy breathing caused by the preceding squats. For a less torturous way to do pullovers, a more traditional 5 sets of 8 reps can also be done with heavier weights than possible after an arduous set of squats.

The key to correctly performing a pullover is to position yourself properly on a sturdy flat bench. Become familiar with how to hold a dumbbell so that you can execute a full range of motion. Fast twitch muscles such as the triceps, lats, pecs, and delts thrive on being stretched with a load and then firing off in full contraction to bring the dumbell to rest above the chest. I am most familiar with the cross bench pullover, although I am aware that you can do a pullover while positioned length wise on a flat bench as well. This position would not allow as great as stretch as the cross bench version during which your hips are lower than your shoulder girdle but it could be a viable option if the lifter cannot into the proper cross bench position.

I myself prefer to complete my pullovers after I press heavily, either flat or incline benches. I have seen lifters be successful training the pullover during a pressing workout, as part of a lat workout or supersetted with breathing squats.

For you aspiring Strongman competitors, a heavy pullover program will allow you to bear hug stones, keep your arch during a heavy yoke or carry, and provide you with the tricep strength to lock out a heavy log over head. For you Jiu Jitsu fighters or wrestlers, having a larger, more muscular torso is advantageous because it makes you harder to take down and nearly impossible to mount due to the fact you will have a torso similar to a grizzly bear.

An analytical look around the landscape of the modern day strength monsters allows one to realize that mega raw benchers such as James Strickland, Matt Wenning, and Eddie Hall all spent their formative years as competitive swimmers. Imagine how many reps they completed with their shoulders and lats going through the full range of motion against medium resistance in the form of water while they trained in swimming. Now, you may not have access to an Olympic size pool to train in, but if you frequent the MF connection then surely you have access to weights. I believe that frequent pullovers can almost mimic some of the training done by swimmers.

A study of the shoulder joint reveals it is the only joint in body that moves through a 360 degree range of motion. The shoulder is designed to move for speed. By training the dumbbell cross bench pullover you are overloading and strengthening this joint in a way that no other exercise can.

I will say that when I began training in the epic Workout Plus Gym in Dedham,

Massachusetts I was able to use an original Nautilus pullover machine which I found as an effective tool but it did not hit my triceps like the cross bench dumbell pullover. Pullover machines take the hands and triceps out of the exercise and therefore are not as effective in stimulating every upper body muscle that the dumbbell version effects.

Recently my sons have taken a much stronger interest in strength training. After one recent workout, my youngest son Max remarked to me that "dumbbell pullovers make him feel better at the end of his workout." That is insightful of my son and also it reminded me that more people should complete exercises that promote their health, specifically in this case the exercise that increases the range of motion in their shoulders while building strength in all of their upper body muscles. When I complete dumbbell pullovers my pecs, both of which I have torn bench pressing, feel great and get stronger with no threat of injury.

Give cross bench dumbbell pullovers a shot at your next workout. Gradually increase your range of motion as you lower the dumbbell behind your head and close to the floor. Allow your joints to get used to the increased range of motion with a weight in your hand. When you pull the bell back over, focus on initiating the lift with your lats and the long head of your tricep as those muscles work in unison to initiate the movement. Position your elbows during the movement so that the most muscle building stress remains in the muscles and not in locked out joints.

Pullovers can totally revamp your physique people. Invest in yourself by engaging in an aggressive dumbbell pullover program and you will soon begin to hope that your favorite style of shirt comes in an XXL size because that is the only thing that will fit your ever growing chest.

Board Press – A History and Practical Application

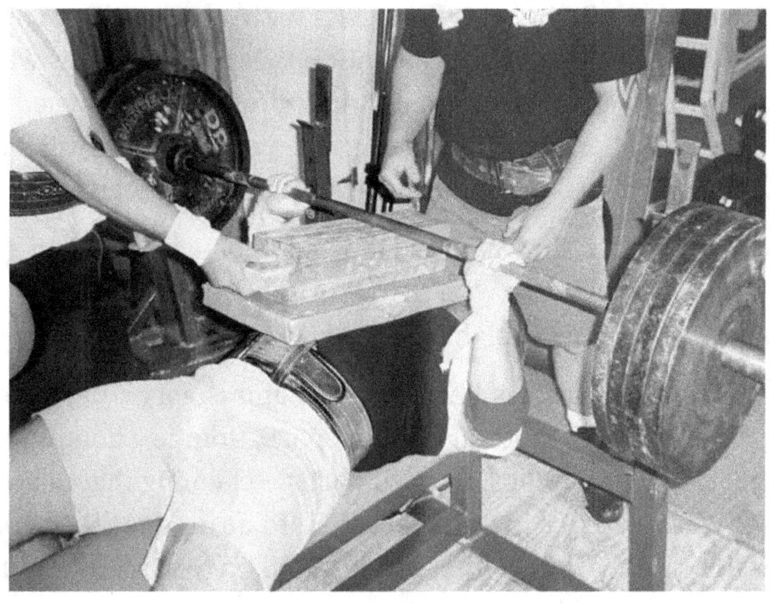

BOARD PRESSING PICTURE CORTESY PAUL LEONARD

The board press is a popular exercise that has been used for over 50 years to improve bench press performance. Originally used by the Culver City Westside crew– the board press was reintroduced to the strength seeking world by Louie Simmons' Columbus Ohio Westside Barbell in the early 1990s. Louie's articles described how his lifters all used board presses to improve their bench presses.

Louie gave full credit to the original Westsiders for coming up with the idea to use board presses to build their benches from various sticking points. On a Powerlifter Video Magazine from 1996, Louie demonstrated how he used 2 x 4s, from 1 to 3 boards placed on the lifters chest. The lifter would take the bar down to however many boards were on the chest- not allowing the bar to sink into the boards too greatly- then pressing the bar from the boards to lockout.

Louie said in that video that he had given up on the board presses years earlier, but Jesse

Kellum convinced Louie to revisit them after Jesse set an all time world record of 602 in the 198 lb class with a bench shirt. Louie explained in the videotape presentation that board presses were part of the 3 to 4 week rotation of max effort exercises used by Westside's best benchers. The max effort method would call for a maximum single to either 1 to 3 boards, using a close grip.

Kenny Patterson is shown on the tape and Louie said he had a 600 lb board press to a board with a close grip- at the smooth of the bar, as well as a 620 press with his pinkie on the ring.

How the board press has been adapted and changed over the years. The first man to total 3000, SuperD Donnie Thompson, who benched over 900lbs, wrote an article claiming that board presses were a great assistance exercise, to be used for 5 sets of 5 reps. He said that short lifters should use up to a three board, while longer armed lifters should use a 4 to 5 board.

A killer variation, triceps death. Super bencher Glen Buchelien was a Westside visitor and disciple who popularized a unique way to use board presses to overload the triceps. What was prescribed was for a lifter to lay on the bench while a spotter would place the one board on the lifters chest- who would then press the bar for 5 reps, at which time the assistant would then rotate a two board onto the lifters chest who would then press the bar for 5 reps, and the assistant would subsequently rotate a 3 board, then a 4 board and finally a 5 board.

The rotating of the boards are to be done as quickly as possible so the set continues without any pause between boards. The goal is to complete 5 presses from 5 different levels as quickly as possible- to overload and stress the fast twitch triceps. Lifters supremely conditioned such as Mike Martin and Glen could then continue from the 5th board back down to the 4 board for 5, then the 3rd board, all the way to the 1 board- for 50 total reps!

Over the years, companies have created products such as **Bench blockz** and shoulder saver pads, which are devices that attach to the bar- mimicking a board press without the need for someone to hold a board on the lifters chest. I feel these are good options and I have used both. There are numerous YouTube videos from the creators of these products that should be helpful.

Like most of Westside Barbell's max effort exercises, board presses could be varied by accommodating resistance modalities such as bands and/or chains affixed to the bar. Although board presses have been associated with shirted bench press training, but in my experience they are useful for raw benchers as well. Matt Wenning, who benched 612 lbs raw, wrote an article how he would bench full range of motion for max effort work one week and then the next he would do board presses the next week for his max effort work, because the pectoral and deltoid tie in do not recover as quickly as the tricep/ lockout phase of the bench. As for myself, after numerous pectoral tears over the years, I have found board presses as a great way to work my bench when my pectorals felt unrecovered.

Board presses can be done with a standard power bar, an axle, a thick squat bar, a parallel grip bar, or any of the bandbell bars made by Louie Simmons old training partner Jimmy Seitzer.

Give board presses a try and I think you will see that they help you build power in your triceps that no other exercise can. This is due to the fact that the limited range of motion leads itself to the use of heavier weights than any other isolation exercise of the triceps.

Shoulder Press Training for Powerlifting and Strongman Success

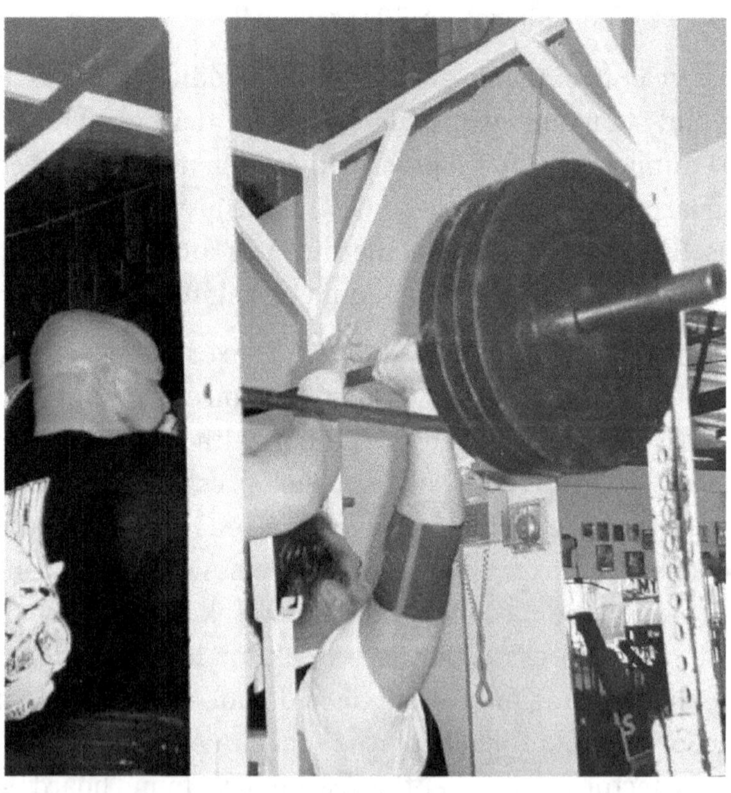

When I began lifting weights in my basement in the early 80s, the shoulder press was one of my favorite lifts. I had to do them seated, but training alone, I always did them because I could push them hard without a spot- if you missed the lift, you just put it back on the bench press uprights on which I was seated.

As soon as I started lifting at my high school for football, I did not focus on any type of military press, until college when I discovered the Bill Kazmaier Muscular Bulk Program, which emphasized shoulder building with standing dumbbell presses and various dumbbell raises. My emphasis was still primarily on the bench press, as I was a powerlifter.

In 1993 I discovered Westside Barbell and Louie Simmons writings. Louie described power rack training among the training principles taught by Anthony Ditillo, a training based author Louie admired who was known for his outrageous muscle mass. The final impactful factor that convinced me to add heavy military presses and power rack presses to my training was a picture of top IFBB Pro Bodybuilder Michael Francois doing 315lb power rack military presses at Westside Barbell!

I had numerous old Ironman Magazines as well as the then current Milo Magazines which had Anthony Ditillo articles in them. I soon purchased Anthony's books, The Development of Muscular Bulk and The Development of Physical Strength. These books were once cited by famous trainer Charles Poliquin as being the best source of training information ever printed. I agree that both of Anthony's books and all of his articles are amazing sources of training information- his books have hundreds of programs, philosophy and some dietary guidelines to follow to gain muscle mass or lose body fat. The only books that I have seen which come close to Ditillo's are those authored by my friend Josh Bryant and Adam Benshea at Jailhouse Strong.

Right as I was lifting a 500lb bench in the gym...my shoulders started to ache and give me problems when I would train. It was

1999 and I decided to add Ditillo style rack military work to my training sessions. I never implemented all of the high volume that Anthony advised in many of his programs, but I certainly used the exercises that he recommended.

For a 6 week period around the holiday season, max Effort bench press night would be replaced with seated partial power rack presses. Often times me and my training partners would work up to a single with the bar resting on a pin level either at our shoulders, chin, nose, or forehead level and lock that out – last man standing! With many strong benchers in my garage gym, we would see many successful attempts of over 300 lbs. When everyone hit their max for the pin level of the day, the pins would be adjusted so that high lockouts, of two inches or so, would be attacked again as a contest between gym members. I know many times I would lock out over 400 lbs.

This workout of power rack military presses was fun, but it also let our shoulders recover from a year of heavy benching. All of us got stronger shoulders from this program. We would take the proper time to warm up and then take our max attempts. When we locked out a press, we would hold the lockout for up to 5 seconds in order to build the rotator cuff as well as tendon and ligaments that make up the shoulder girdle- the only joint in the body that rotates 360 degrees. Make sure you are firmly seated on a bench or military press bench- with lower back support. Take a shoulder width grip and squeeze the bar hard. I would pull down on the bar to begin my single attempts- in order to activate my rotator cuff muscles prior to pushing up to lockout out the bar.

Look at any strength great who pushed their shoulder press up to world class level and you will see that the presses built all three heads of their deltoids and the resulting muscular development could not be achieved without such presses. I am talking about Bill Kazmaier, **Ted Arcidi, Zydrunas Savickas, Eddie Hall,** or Josh Bryant. Military presses are the safest way to build the strongest shoulders in the world! All these lifters did some lateral raises and front raises, but the bulk of their shoulder training was presses.

We would always work up to heavy singles in the power rack military presses- but there were workouts where we would finish with pump sets of 225 for 20 reps on the two inch lockout or even 135 for 20 on the presses from the shoulder, neck or chin level. The flushing of blood leaks felt therapeutic. Pumping up your shoulders is a very effective method of training, one that was also written about by the first man to bench 600lbs raw, Pat Casey.

After a few months for the power rack military press program, I would suggest the lifter transition to full range of motion standing military presses with a Barbell or a pair of dumbbells. Shoulders recover quicker than chest muscles, so a lifter can train their shoulder presses at least twice per week. Recall that the top Olympic lifters of the 1970s like Vasily Alekseyev and Ken Patera had military presses of over 500 lbs by pressing frequently with low reps and many sets.

To correctly do a standing press, take a shoulder width grip on a bar loaded on a rack, take a deep breath and unrack the bar, stepping back to take a firm, shoulder width stance- toes gripping the floor and heels locked down. Now take another deep breath, hold it, and press the bar over the head while fully locking the arms out with the elbows in line with the ears of the lifter. Pause for a second- having exhaled your breath as the toughest part of the lift. Inhale as you lower the bar and re-set for another repetition. I preferred sets of 5 reps for the full range of motion military presses and higher repetitions for the dumbbell presses- Kaz recommended 10 rep sets!

Did this program work? I would not be writing about it if it did not. In 1999, I was stuck at a 470 lb bench with achy shoulders- to benching 534 in 2000 to beat the great Josh Bryant at the National Championships. When I began competing in strongman. I pressed a 275lb log for 3 reps and also did push press of 320 at the U.S.

Strongest Man Contest in 2005. And speaking of Josh, he did plenty heavy rack presses en route to his push press of 445 to win the U.S. Strongest Man title.

Zercher Squat – A Beautifully Brutal Exercise

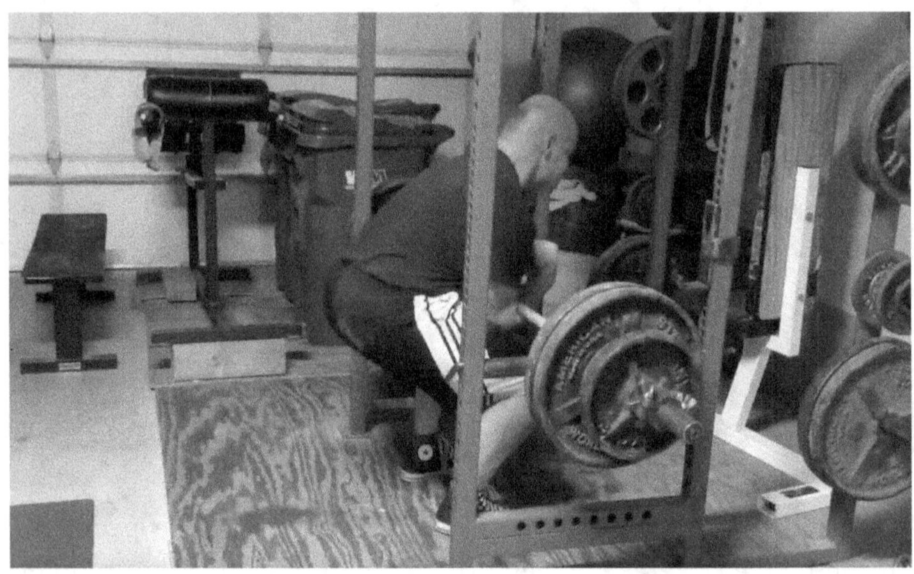

I first learned about the zercher squat from Louie Simmons of the Westside Barbell in Columbus, Ohio. Ed Zercher of Missouri invented this lift. Louie described how this old school lift was done out of necessity by an inmate Robert Barnett, who was incarcerated and therefore had no access to a squat or any type of rack. To build his body, Mr. Barnett would squat down to the bar loaded on the ground and then he would place his bent arms under the bar and squat it off the ground.

Louie Simmons said that for larger lifters who were bulkier and lacked the flexibility to lift the bar off the ground, then a variation would be to take the bar from a power rack while in the crook of your elbows and squat down below parallel. Louie said he had done a best lift of 500lbs in an exhibition in this style. This became my goal!

I found that this exercise made me very strong, if I worked up to a maximum single as a max effort exercise. I was eventually able to work up to a strong 550lb single with a belt that was at parallel and I tried a 585 that I stood up with, but I did not go that deep. The Zercher squat is responsible for my PR squat of 810, 750 conventional deadlift, and all the strongman competition lifts I did with stones over 300 lbs to platforms as well as flipping an 800lb tire.

How I performed the Zercher Squat:

I would set a Texas power bar in the J-cups outside the power rack, so that I could squat down and take the bar into to the crooks of my elbow and walk back to clear the rack and take my stance. I would set up wide enough with my feet so that when I squatted down, my elbows would lightly scrape my knees on the inside and I would hit parallel. My goal was always the same, to lower myself under control so that my hips were lower than they would be at the start of my conventional stance deadlift. I would then stand back up and lock the weight out. I experimented with reps up to 5, but nothing got me as strong a heavy ass singles.

I would wear a belt and chalk the inside of my elbows to prevent bar slippage. I never did a Zercher squat to a box, nor did I use bands, chains or pauses when doing this type of squat. This was the beautiful simplicity of this exercise- just focus on squatting as deep and under control as you can- locking out the weight, holding it for a second at lockout and then returning it to the rack.

Zercher squats, what they built on me:

Zercher squats made my abdominal muscles stronger than any exercise I ever trained. They built my posterior chain, with the weight in front of my hips, they stressed my hips and hamstrings- which are hip extenders. I felt that they made my lower back feel better if it was a bit tired or over trained. As important as physical conditioning and strengthening, the mental benefits I got from Zercher squats were just as important to me. As the first man to total 2500, 2600, 2700, 2800, and 2900...Gary Frank always said you had to become "bear wrasslting" strong. He was right! For me, taking a quarter of a ton into my arms and squatting it up and back tightened "my mental screws", as the late, great Dr. Ken Leistner wrote. Working in law enforcement for over 30 years, I love to be aggressive in the gym and Zercher squats make me feel powerful and required a brutal focus.

Other exercises I trained with Zercher squats:

I would do Zercher squats after doing dynamic effort deadlifts, the Westside program of 15 singles with 65%, 12 singles with 70%, 10 singles with 75%, 8 singles with 80%, 6 singles with 85%, pull a maximum on the 6th week and repeat. At times, I would do Zercher squats to begin a workout and couple them with kneeling squats. I was a great kneeling squatter, able to do 900 for 1, there is an Instagram post of me Zercher squatting 450 and then doing 785 for 6 kneeling squats. I often did heavy side bends when I did Zercher squats, my gym in California had dumbbells to 225 and I would go that heavy for sets of 5 reps per side.

Another exercise I found very useful to combine with Zercher squats is pull throughs with a cable. Because I Zercher squatted with a medium width stance, I would do cable pull throughs with my squat stance or a foot width wider. The cable stack I used went up to 400 lbs, but sets with approximately 220 to 280 was great for sets of 10 reps to really build my hamstrings.

Other lifters who I know Zercher squatted more than I did/do:

With the creation of YouTube, I was able to see some great lifters who used the Zercher squat to build strength and power. Strongman legend Nick Best can be seen lifting 705 on the lift! Kevin Oak has a clip of a 605 Zercher squat. Many of today's MMA and Jiu Jitsu champions, such as Phil Daru can be seen online training and programming the Zercher squat. I do too for the fighters and football players I train.

Give the Zercher your best effort and I know you will be stronger and mentally tougher for excelling at this lift.

Squatting to SUPER Low Boxes, Milk Crates, Hassocks and Cinder Blocks

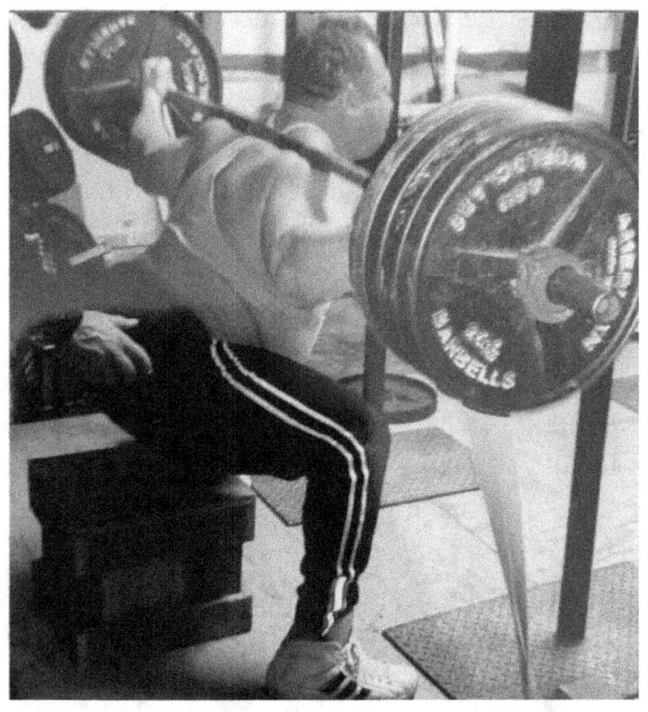

I began training my squat via the <u>Westside Barbell</u> Box Squat training program in 1994. The staple in my program was the 12" box, which guaranteed that every repetition I did on the squat was below parallel. As Louie Simmons instructed, if every rep in training is below parallel, you will never have to ask your buddies if you squatted deep enough.

Louie Simmons had written about squatting to a hassock as early as 1988 in Powerlifting USA, but I did not follow his advice then. I obtained a hassock and added it to my routine. By the time I began box squatting, I had a best official squat of 615 lbs, so I was an intermediate level lifter. I had suffered a hip injury goofing around at a pool so I started squatting to a milk crate that was 10" high.

My training routine at the time was the standard 12 sets of 2 reps for two weeks, then 10 sets of 2 reps on Dynamic Effort lower body night. These squats were done with my competition stance and to a 12" box. This workout could be best called "ten minutes of terror" as I would race the clock to do all the sets in two AC DC songs. There was no sitting down between sets. This workout was the three week dynamic wave for which the poundage percentages were 50, 55 and 60 % of my contest maximum for the 12 or 10 doubles. There was no accommodating resistance with bands or chains used- but I did follow Louie's advice and try to do each repetition with as much force as possible- Fred Hatfield's Compensatory Acceleration. After the week of 10 doubles at 60 % you would begin the wave over at 50%.

At times, I would then squat to the milk crate for 8 to 10 singles with as wide as I could stand and pause on the crate. The idea was the extreme range of motion and the loaded bar would strengthen my hip joints. This worked perfectly as my hips healed and I put 100lbs on my total each year for 5 years. I never used more than 225, 245, or 275 for these squats, but I learned that squatting extremely low to an object was a great way for me to get stronger. Why so many sets of squats? As Louie said, they did a lot of a few things at Westside. I was hungry to build a new base of strength and squatting for over 20 sets per workout on DE was the price I paid to eventually squat 810 and stand up easily with 859 at the Nationals, to lose the call on depth.

As for the hassock squat, initially, I would use the squat to the hassock as a max effort exercise with a closer than competition stance. I would vary the height of the hassock by placing a 45 or 100lb plate under the hassock. Once I could squat 500lbs and pause it on the foam hassock, my competition squat went to

700lbs. This exercise also increased my leg strength for starting deadlifts.

In my training experience, super low box squats made me very strong without wearing out my nervous system or my body. There are many reasons for this, first 500 lbs to a 12" or less boss is less stressful than handling 700 plus pounds on the squat to a parallel position. When you handle heavy squat weight, it takes a toll on your shoulders and arms- specifically the elbow/brachialis region on the forearms. This makes heavy bench pressing difficult during a training week. The positive carry over from deep box squats allowed me to do less deadlifting and avoid Central Nervous System burnout that comes from too much deadlifting.

As I got stronger as the three lift powerlifter that I wanted to become, I learned to optimize my training efforts so that each lift received the proper amount of training and one lift's training did not negatively impact another lift.

As I got stronger with my squat, I added squatting to a side by side set of cinder blocks. I did this movement because after box squatting for a few years, my quads lagged behind my hamstrings and hips strength. At 6'2", narrow stance squats to cinder blocks built quads. I would vary the height of the cinder blocks with 1/2" wood sheets on top.

My training was done in my garage and I had no fancy equipment to target quads such as a leg press, hack squat machine or belt squat set up. The cinder squat worked great and allowed me to compete in powerlifting and strongman for 20 plus years after mastering it. My training partners also used the cinder block squat as well as various box squats to become some of the best competitive squatters of their time and class.

 My one time protege, Josh Bryant, one upped all his Yorba Barbell mentors with a 700 squat to a 9" cube- as seen on YouTube. I eventually built up to some awesome weights, for me, on low boxes and hassocks. Many of those lifts are on my Paul L YouTube Channel as well my **Instagram**.

Knowing what I know now, deep box squats can be used with bands, chains, specialty bars and the lightened method as well. As Super D, Donnie Thompson says, to add to the horror you could squat with kettlebell, fat bells, a keg or a sandbag to a low box- as shown by Brad Gillingham on his HMB blog lately.

Give super deep object squats your best effort and let me know how they work for you.

HISTORY MATTERS Westside Barbell – The History of the Ohio version under Louie Simmons

The original Westside Barbell was created in Culver City, California in the early 1960s by a man named Bill "Peanuts" West. West was a fixture at Muscle Beach in Santa Monica and later Venice Beach. He lived in Culver City, California which is near Venice on the west side of the Los Angeles metropolitan area. West's garage on Neosho became the first Westside Barbell with famous members such as George Frenn and Pat Casey- the first powerlifting legends as well as pioneers.

Thankfully for every powerlifter today, publisher Joe Weider had the vision to include powerlifting information in his magazine, Muscle Builder Power. The training methods and successes of the Westside Culver Crew was promoted around the globe and in Germany, at an army base, a young U.S. soldier named Louis Simmons read these magazines and it heavily influenced his thinking and most importantly his training. Louie returned to Columbus, Ohio and became a national level powerlifter. Louie has said on many occasions that his first training partners were a power rack, an AM radio, and a mirror in his basement gym. On many of Louie's podcast and in his excellent book, the Iron Samurai, Louie details how he partnered initially with Tom Palluci, Jimmy

Seitzer, and Doug Heath after meeting them at the Ohio State weight room.

Louie incorporated and trademarked the name Westside Barbell in 1987- recently relating how thrilled he was to get a telephone call from George Frenn- whom he idolized, even though Frenn demanded $5,000 dollars for Louie's use of the name Westside Barbell. Louie has always detailed how the original Westside lifters and their articles opened his eyes to box squatting, bench lockouts, incline presses, board presses, and touch deadlifts – all feature articles in the late 1960s Muscle Builder Power magazines and available today in Dave Yarnel's excellent book; "The lost secrets of the Original Westside Barbell." Louie's free articles on his website always detail where and from whom Louie learned a strength gaining tactic.

In the late 80s, Louie wrote articles for Powerlifting USA magazine and although I read them, I did not understand or apply his theories. At that time, Louie was retired from lifting and was known for his wife Doris' lifting as well as females Laura Dodd, Debbie Sorenson and Susie Benford. Jeff Chorpenning was a National champion who appeared in PLUSA with crazy pictures of him doing sit ups with 315 on the decline bench at Lou's gym. Matt Dimmel was the most famous powerlifter associated with Westside Barbell, but when he competed he would wear a Black's Health World shirt and he represented that famous gym out of Cleveland, Ohio.

Much like the original Westside in Culver City had an instate rival gym, Zuvers, Westside Ohio had Black's Health World and Larry Pacifico's Power Crew in Dayton, Ohio to push their performance.

Louie described in recent podcasts and YouTube interviews that he opened a commercial gym in the late eighties and it was there that he met Chuck Vogelpohl, Kenny Patterson and some of his other members who would remain as Louie described: "Westsiders for life."

Westside Barbell garnered international fame based upon their lifters success as well as from their articles in Powerlifting USA, which was accompanied by advertisements for their video tape instructional series for each lift. These ads started appearing in 1993, which was when I bought them. They changed my lifting life entirely and I have, in the spirit of Louie Simmons, done my best to pass on what I have learned from the system. Louie's writings soon appeared in Milo, which was the premiere strength training journal in the US from 1993 until it ceased publication in 2018. Louie also appeared numerous times on Powerlifter video magazine to teach and he also released another half a dozen video tapes/dvds with priceless training wisdom. Within ten years of the release of the original tapes in 1993, Westside lifters dominated the top geared powerlifting meets in the United States such as the World

Powerlifting Organization (WPO), which was contested primarily at the Arnold

Schwarzenegger Classic Exposition in Columbus, Ohio as well as at other fitness exposition.

As Westside's popularity increased, many internet websites and messages boards were focused on discussing and analyzing the Westside system.

As the internet developed, Westside launched and maintains a great website today. There are many Westside Barbell YouTube videos online as well as lifters and athletes who follow the system. Instagram and Facebook has had Westside based content for the better part of a decade. There is also a fantastic documentary called Westside vs the World on the streaming platform Netflix.

I thoroughly enjoy and learn from Louie's podcasts which provide invaluable information. Much like the gym has evolved, so has the way in which the training and information learned by the gym is shared, provided and sold, as today there are numerous downloadable pieces of content you can buy from their website as well as certification programs which you can access and complete.

Venice Beach – The Second Golden Era Of The 1990s

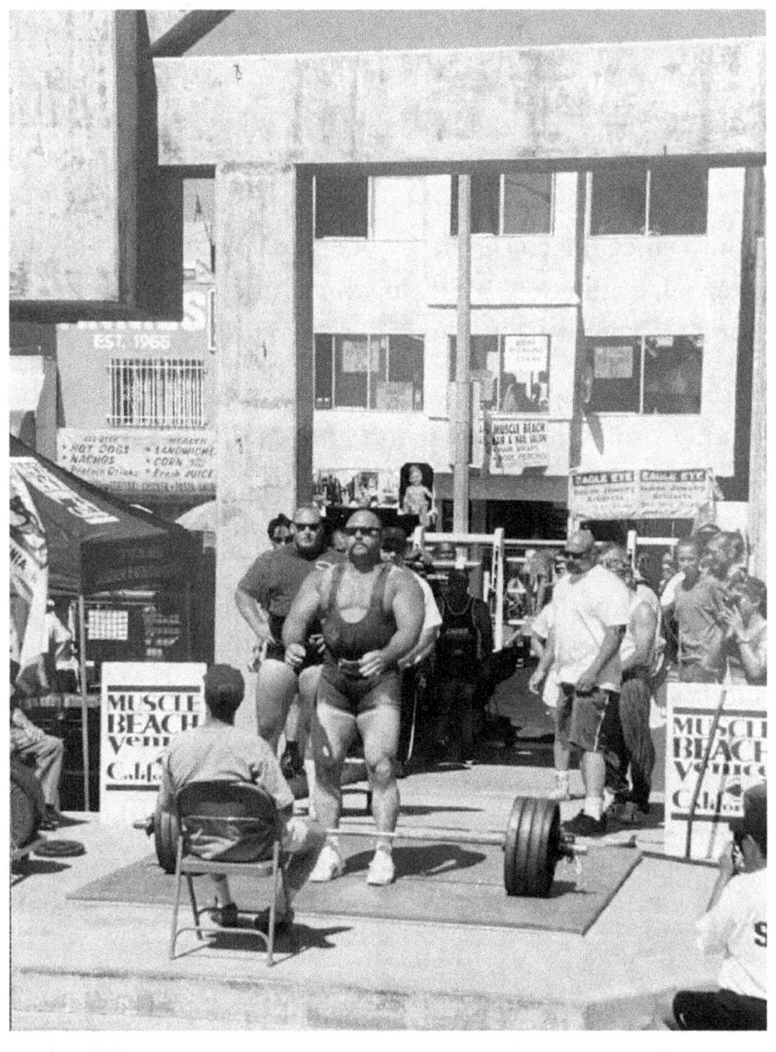

I would assume that anyone who reads this site has seen the documentary Pumping Iron, which details that training of top bodybuilders at Golds Gym in Venice Beach in the mid 1970s, which today is referred to nostalgically as the Golden Age. This documentary was mandatory viewing for those of us who started lifting in the 80s, because frankly there was not much else other than muscle magazines- which were also gold in the seventies through the eighties. Everyone had a copy of this movie on VHS and it was must see viewing before heading to the Y or whatever real gym you trained at. After watching the training scenes a few hundred times and seeing Arnold living in So California like a fucking boss, this Bostonian's mind was made up-I would live in California one day. During house parties in high school, MTV would be on and whenever the Gap Band's Party Train played, I would watch the Venice Beach themed video and say-I will be there some day. After all, in the 80s, Hulk Hogan claimed he was from Venice Beach upon his entrance to the squared circle.

In 1991, I moved to Los Angeles two weeks after I graduated college to begin my professional life. Soon after arriving, I made my first trip to Venice a Beach one day. I was disappointed to see that the weight pen area was closed and boarded up for renovations. I went over to check out Golds Gym and before getting in the door, I was met by bodybuilder Paul Dillet-whom I recognized from the muscle mags of the day. Paul acted as if he recognized me and then told me he could not find his car. I offered to help him and I was shocked that he was paranoid, confused, and incoherent at times- mumbling and not making any sense. I have no idea what was running through his system, but I wanted none of it and a few years later when he was close to one of the best bodybuilders on earth I shook my head. Maybe everything written in those magazines was not exactly the truth about healthy living and dedication to training.

I returned to Venice a few more times that summer as it was cool to people watch. I was down to my last bit of saved money prior to getting a real job, but I do fondly recall spending my last 100 dollar bill in the Ironman Magazine Store buying the old Peary Rader edition of the magazine with black and white print and great information from Anthony Ditillo and the strength stars of the time. These magazines were in mint condition and the clueless clerk sold them for $ 1 dollar an issue because " no one wants any magazine without chicks in it or not in color." I still have these issues today.

For that price I was able to buy a decade and a half of value as the original Ironman came out with only 6 issues per year.

I got my career started and did not visit Venice again for two years until I was ready to compete there. I am writing this piece on one of my favorite days of the year, the first day of summer, or the solstice. Today is the longest day of the year, so an Irish/German mutt such as myself can appreciate a day when you can get the most work in due to it's length.

As a strength athlete living in Southern California during the 90s through the mid 2000s, the beginning of summer meant one great thing-frequent lifting meets at the Venice Beach Weight pen. Powerlifting USA would publish a list of upcoming contests and the USPF Powerlifting meet schedule would include bench press, deadlift, and push pull meets at the famed Venice Beach. State Powerlifting chair, promoter extraordinaire, and helluva of powerlifter himself Steve Dennison would always schedule meets in Venice. I recall that there was a woman named Darlene Galindo, Joe Wheatley, and Kevin Meskew were responsible for organizing and then running these Powerlifting and odd lift meets such as the Iron Warrior Strongman Challenge as well as frequent curl meets. Every strength related contest was MC'd by the incredibly talented Chuck Lamantia.

In June of 1993 I competed in the Venice Beach Deadlift Open and won the 275lb class with a pull of 660lbs. At the time, I had been training at American Eagle Gym in Norwalk California with powerlifters named CT Fletcher, Richard Schoenberger, and Steve Winslow.

The American Eagle was a cool little gym, I believe still open, and run by the nice Sherry Houston. The best thing about the Venice meet was that I met up with Gary Hogan and he invited me to train with he and his crew- which I soon did beginning in 1995. During 1994, I trained solo and began implementing the Westside Barbell System. As Louie Simmons has said, at times my only training partners were a power rack, a radio, and the info from the muscle magazines of the day. Louie had Muscle Builder Power with the Original Culver City Westside material, I had Milo, PLUSA, and the bodybuilding based magazines of the day.

Although I had won at Venice in 1993, I kept reading about these alleged powerlifters at Golds Gym in Venice that we're getting lots of publicity in Musclemag International and Muscular Development who were so much stronger than what myself or anyone from Gary's crew was. The names Mike O'hearn, Elder, and Fedkiw kept being repeated as forces to be dealt with on the platform. At about the same time, PLUSA began publishing a column by Ned Low called PowerScene that extolled the performances of the Golds based powermen.

Ned, who became my friend, also created and distributed the Powerlifter Video Magazine VHS tapes during that time frame which initially promoted any lifter from Golds Venice. This fueled my fire and I would later see, it fueled Art Labare and Gary Hogan's as well.

The 1995 USPF California State meet was a turning point in my Powerlifting career. I lost to Steve Dennison but I out totaled Mike O'hearn and no one from Gold's Venice impressed at the biggest State meet California had for years before or for the following ten years. I will do

a separate entire article on the 95 State meet, with the meet's video footage included, at a later date. But following this meet, the aura of any Powerlifter, other than the amazing Ron Fedkiw, was off any of the Venice guys.

By 1996, Art, Ric Purchase, Brian Meek, and myself would circle National and World level meets on the Calendar as our targets for the coming year. Other affiliated Yorba members such as Ron Perkins, Mike Morgan, Ray Cosio, Al Morentin, George Pessel, and Gary Garcia would compete at local meets- to include Venice.

Venice always had a special place in our hearts and chip on our collective shoulder as we went there to kick in opposing lifters teeth on the platform. Professional wrestling television ratings wars at the time had the NWO Wolfpack pitted against Degeneration X. Yorba acted and performed like we were Big Poppa Pump and Kevin Big Sexy Nash as opposed to the Golds crew who were the crotch grabbing, 16" armed Shawn, got my ass kicked by construction workers in real life, Michaels. Venice became our playground and we were certain to go compete there regularly. Like Louie Simmons says, always compete locally, even if you are a national caliber athlete, in order to grow the sport.

Competing in Venice was different because the warm up area left a lot to, be desired and being in the sun all day ended up being a bit more draining. No wonder Arnold napped in it.

In addition to my buddies, there were so many great lifters who competed or were present at Venice in those times. CT Fletcher and Rich Schoenberger benched huge, Larry Horton pulled huge weights, and the final meet I attended at Venice saw Scott Mendelson bench 876 lbs in the summer of 2003.

I was there with my oldest son Lou on my shoulders. He clung on real tight when I stopped to bullshit with Andrew Brynarski- who was as huge as ever and must have looked frightening when he was in his Leatherface costume. That was the year they remade Texas Chainsaw Massacre and Andy at times I think liked that character a bit much.

Andy was not the biggest human I ever saw in person at Venice, that would be then professional bodybuilder Chris Duffy-who was hanging out with then Ironman writer Lonnie Tepper. Except for Rory Leidelmeyer, I have only seen one other bodybuilder who was bigger in person-Greg Kovacs. I have no comment on Chris Duffy's other identity or his life choicesI can just tell you when I met him he was enormous, as in small planets should be circling him.

During that same time period, I would travel to Venice to visit often. In the late 90s within a few miles radius of Gold's Gym there was World Gym (RIP-now it is a residence! Arnold should own it), Powerhouse Gym, and the Marina Athletic Club-where famous pictures of Dorian being trained by Mike Metzner were shot.

Only Gold's survives today. To eat in the area, the Firehouse was great with many bodybuilders present, but we also used to eat at Schatzi's on main. This place was Arnold's restaurant and it was great food and had lots of pretty people to see. Picture a nice place to eat brunch, open, airy, with a huge dude every 20 feet wearing a red Hawaiian shirt- but serving as a host? Say what you will but Arnold always gave jobs to bodybuilders and wannabes. One of these host was a Vietnamese guy named Bingo Binh who was about 5'8" 300lbs with 20 plus inch calves. The other was Michael Clark Duncan (RIP) from the Green Mile.

What about training in Venice? I could have cared less after beating Mike O'hearn in 95. The mystique was gone. My garage was full of the best powerlifters in Southern California. Ned Low drove out to my garage to film an episode of Powerlifter Video Magazine and to write up my gym in PLUSA.

I did train at Golds one more time. It was a Saturday evening in 95 and with my girl out of town, I thought let me see what this Gold's has. First off, of the 3 rooms it was then- no 100lb plates. None. Well in any commercial gym my default workout is always upper back- how can you screw that up. I was training at about 6 pm and the gym was mostly deserted except for a very well built lady who was repping 185 on the bench for sets of 10.

She came over to me at one point and asked me if I would spot her. I said sure thing. She had 135 on the bar at this point. I handed off and she took it down and the bar did not leave her chest. She asked for a spot so I upright the bar and replaced it. She then told me I spotted her wrong, she needed forced reps. I tried to do a traditional forced rep for her but she exclaimed no! She then proceeded to flip my hands around so my palms were facing down and then said like this. She unracked the bar and took it down easily under control with my hands between the bar and her chest. Once my hands were on her implants she tried to move enticingly or sexy in her mind and she moaned and said yes. Too weird for me so I re-racked the bar and said no way. I figured out then that is why the Gold's guys weren't beating us- too many distractions.

I loved competing at Venice as well as supporting my friends there when they layed it on the line. I would look forward to lining up weigh ins to see who I would be up against that day- but the greatest challengers were always from my garage. It was just much funner for us to do it "where the sun meets the sand, where Arnold and Franco got a tan."

I never lifted in a meet against Mike O'hearn again. Trust me I tried and entered them. In California, in Venice, as well as National ones in Chicago and Pennsylvania. As I understand it, I heard he was busying modeling. Well two can play at that game. If you look at the 2002 Muscle Beach brochure- there I am in between attempts, supporting my man Art as we kicked some more Venice Beach teeth in.....guess Mike was booked that day....

I moved to Texas in 2004 and have not been back to Venice Beach since. Sadly the competitions run there by Steve Denison and Chuck Lamantia are no more. In 2018 former World Strongest Man competitor Tom Magee was severely beaten by 6 men over a parking spot dispute. World Gym is now a private residence and the area is surrounded by homeless encampments. I am so glad I got to enjoy Venice during it's second golden era of the 1990s.

Powerlifting Gyms and Clubs – A History of Where Many Strength Legends Began

When I began Powerlifting, I was gifted with a complete collection of Powerlifting USA Magazines, which began publication in 1977. Fortunately for me, many of the authors for the magazine, such as Dr. Ken Leistner, Marty Gallagher, Mike Lambert, Ron Fernando and Louie Simmons had a strong sense of the history of the sport and shared it with their readers. I immediately realized that many of the great lifters of the past were part of Powerlifting clubs that laid the foundation for future clubs and a culture that breeds strength success.

The first Powerlifting club discussed was the Original Westside Barbell Club of Culver City California that was established by Bill "Peanuts" West in the mid 1960s. Powerlifting Hall of Fame members Pat Casey and George Frenn, as well as many of the strength stars of that era trained at Westside. Thankfully, Armand Tanny chronicled their training exploits for then Joe

Weider's Muscle Builder Power Magazine. Dr. Ken Leistner traveled to and trained at Westside Barbell and detailed his experiences and knowledge in multiple articles.

Dr. Ken also trained at the contemporary rival Powerlifting club of the time as well, Zuvers in Costa Mesa, California. Dr. Ken's articles describing the unique atmosphere of Zuvers are famous in the hardcore Powerlifting world. Thorbecke's in the Phoenix area created many successful champions, notably the immortal Jon Cole and Jack Barnes, yet their training and club culture was not put in print even a fraction as much as Westside and Zuvers.

Dr. Ken and Tanny's articles described how the training environment at both Westside and Zuvers resulted in both clubs producing world record performances in many of their lifters. This led me to be convinced that I needed to find a powerlifting club if I wanted to achieve my strength goals.

I left my local YMCA and found Workout Plus in Dedham, Massachusetts in 1987. Workout plus was a huge fitness center that was the creation of Dick Paaso, a University of Oklahoma Football player whose vision was a place where every member of the community could train, yet he loved heavy training and powerlifting. After a year of training hard, supporting the advanced powerlifters on the gym's team, I was granted admission to the team. The requirements were that I had to compete at least at State level competitions, I had be a great teammate and I was expected to work at any of our own gym's sanctioned contests.

It was at Workout Plus that I learned the culture of Powerlifting, how to correctly spot a lifter, how to load a bar, how to take care of the gym's equipment, how to train, and most importantly how to be respectful of every gym member- regardless of their strength or fitness goals. While learning those skills, I was granted a yearly free membership for myself and a training partner of my choice, meet entry reimbursement, branded attire and a great bunch of grown men who had my back and always helped me with many of life's problems.

During the Eighties while I was training, Powerlifting USA covered teams at Samsons in Orange, California, Black's Healthworld of Cleveland, Ohio, Westside Barbell of Columbus, Ohio, Frantz of Naperville, Illinois and the Wild Bunch in West Virginia. There were other clubs, such as Suncoast in Florida, as well as the Thompson Power Team of Southern California. Not as much was written about the culture of those clubs, but many of their lifters performances spoke volumes.

Louie Simmons wrote articles on his clubs training philosophy and Frantz wrote a fantastic book about powerlifting called his Ten Commandments. I relocated to Southern California to begin my professional career in 1991. Between 91 and 94, I trained at The American Eagle Gym in Norwalk, California as well as PowerHouse Gym of Chatsworth. The Eagle was home to Richard Schoenberger and CT Fletcher, two amazing bench pressers- as well as great men, but neither gym had an established powerlifting club.

During this time, Westside Barbell released this famous video tape series and had a monthly column in Powerlifting USA Magazine, as it had become the most famous powerlifting club in the world. I joined a gym called Uptown Gym in Whittier, California in 1995- becoming a member of their powerlifting crew, which taught me a lot and helped me become stronger.

How I established my own Powerlifting Club

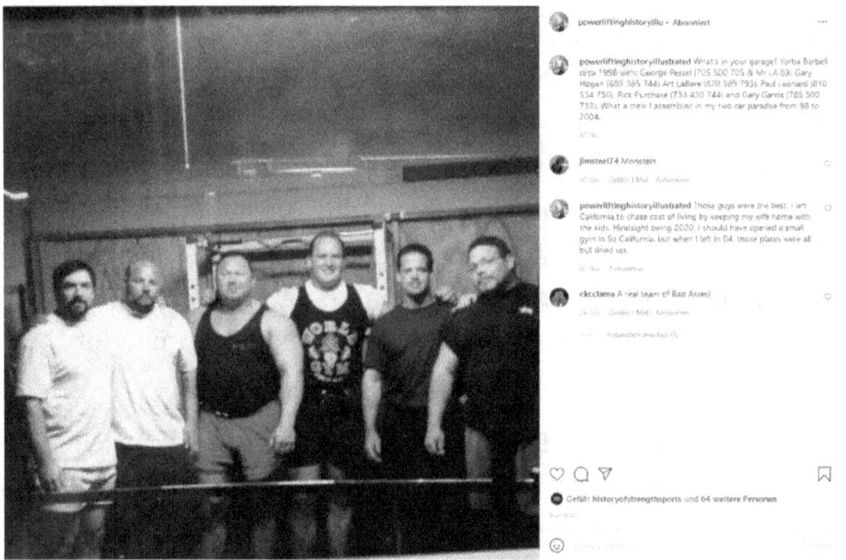

Note: Old

Footages of Yorba barbell are available on Paul's Youtube Channel. Here's the link : [Yorba Barbell Youtube](#)

Despite having a good crew and a decent gym, I was determined to have my own gym at a house I purchased in 1996. The house had a two car garage, which I slowly converted to a gym for two years, at which time in late 1997, I opened Yorba Barbell, in Yorba Linda, California. By competing in Southern California meets since 1993, I had identified and made friends with all the strong Powerlifters that would be my teammates. I came in 2nd at the 1995 California State Championship, won the best lifter trophy at a 1996 local meet and my performances had established me as a serious lifter. Thankfully, there were no better powerlifting club options in Orange County, California in 1997 so my garage became the "go to spot."

Lessons I had learned along the way were to buy the best equipment possible, train as hard as possible, and be positive and honest with my teammates about form, squat depth and training issues. Keep the gym clean, have a great sound system, and always recruit strong, high character people to come to train. Everyone who trained at my gym competed and if you didn't enter the contest, you went to support any member of our club who was competing. At meets, you were expected to wear the team's T-shirt and be a recruiter as well as an ambassador of the club. If some local lifter was really good at a certain lift or had improved greatly since the last meet- find out what they were doing in training and where they were doing it.

I remember how excited I was to buy equipment for my gym. I bought wood from Home Depot to build the platform and horse stall mats from the local feed store for other areas of my garage floor. I bought a brand new **Body Solid power rack** from an exercise store in Yorba Linda for 179 dollars. This rack held up to 900 lbs on many occasions. This rack is still used by my good friend Mike Martin in Texas today. There was a local publication in Southern California called the Pennysaver that was like **Craig's list**-it had an exercise equipment section where I found people selling gym equipment and weights.

In the fall of 1997, I saw an ad for a Golds Gym that was closing in the Inland Empire, about 45 minutes from my house. I got there, drinking my Ford Escort, a compact car, and I met a gym broker who was there already and had bought most of the equipment.

The gym broker, whom I believe was named Larry, was a shrewd businessman- but appreciated my passion, intensity and 300lb frame. He sold me 10 awesome American Worldclass Barbell plates that were made in California during the 1960s. I bought a Barbell that is a clone of a **Texas power bar**, a flat bench, and a military press bench – all for 400 dollars. I still have all this equipment today.

The final thing I bought that day was a pair of 130lb dumbbells-which Larry said he would charge me 10 dollars, if I could carry them farmers walk style to my car. I was up to the challenge and have those great dumbbells today. I jammed all of this equipment into my Escort, making the tires look lower, and I drove it home. This equipment started my gym and I then added more pieces gradually, as I didn't have much money then for lifting, but I got what I needed and we immediately started to get stronger together.

In Southern California my gym members were Art LaBare, Gary Hogan, Gary Garcia, George Pessel, Brian Meek, Ric Purchase, Kevin Kinzy, Charley Kaptur, and the legend Josh Bryant.

Buy nice shirts and attire for your lifters. Hang out with them outside the gym. My training partners and I shared many meals, trips, laughs and adventures together. If your training and gym environment is not fun and making you better- find another gym or club.

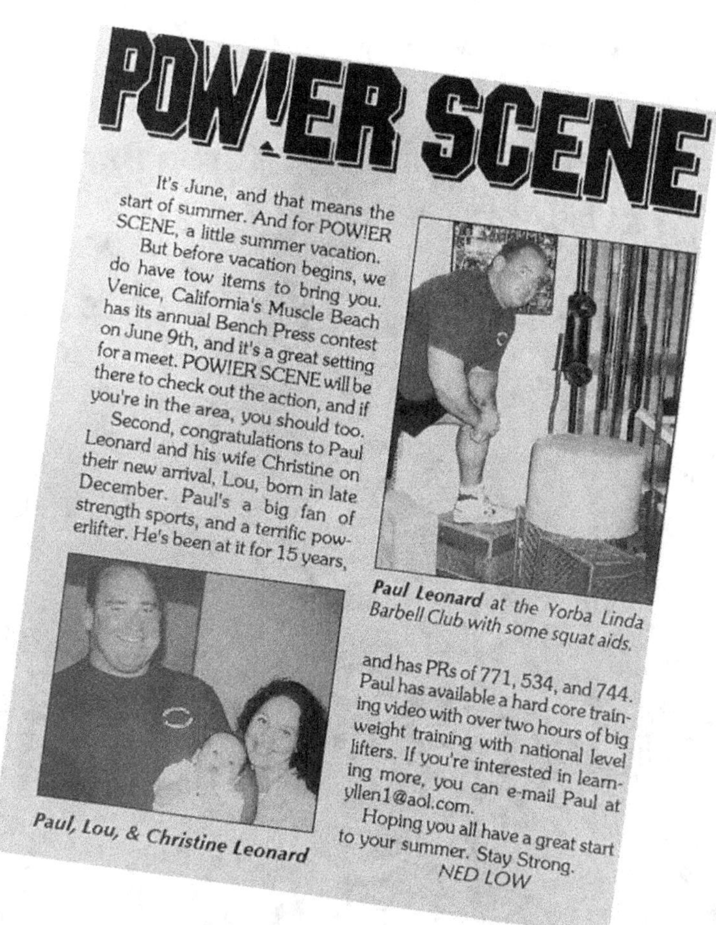

Paul Leonard at the Yorba Linda Barbell Club with some squat aids.

Paul, Lou, & Christine Leonard

Read and research strength training all the time when you run a club. Promote your lifters all the time. There was no social media in the early 2000s, but I used powerlifting message boards and PLUSA Magazine to promote my club and sell a video tape of us training hard- thanks to Dr. Ken Leistner. Today with social media, always promote your fellow lifters and club. I do that today with Beaststrong Powerhouse in Tucson. I had to relocate from Southern California to Texas for work in 2004, but I have always maintained a gym in my garage. I have trained with competitive lifters in Texas and now in Arizona. Often times I teach correct powerlifting and strongman club culture and etiquette to new lifters. I have a blast watching new lifters get strong and learn the beauty that is a successful powerlifting club.

The Training Philosophy at Yorba Barbell

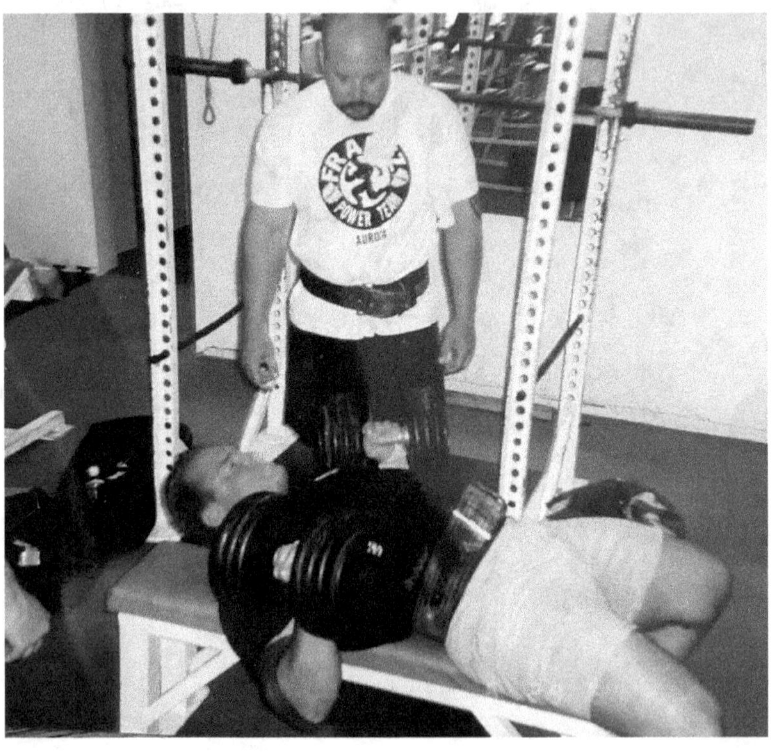

I founded Yorba Barbell in 1997 when I turned my two car garage into a gym. I had been following Westside Barbell/ Louie Simmons' training system based upon his video tapes and published articles. Although I had been invited to Westside, I never went. I began sharing the platform with some of their stars in 1996 and although they impressed me- I am a student of the game so I realize many others had gotten very strong without following Westside principles.

Fortunately for me, I lived in Southern California- arguably the birthplace of powerlifting where many of the legends still lived. Louie Simmons has said many times that he was heavily influenced by the Original Westside Barbell Club of Southern

California. Louie had also described how he was jealous that Roger Estep had been able to travel to Southern California in the late 70s and he went from a 1600lb total in Ohio to a 1900lb world record total in California under the tutelage of Westside founder George Frenn. How lucky was I, that as I became friends with Art LaBare, I found out that Roger was Art's mentor and lived nearby. Two other mentors of Art are Terry McCormick and Dave Shaw. These men, who trained Bill Kazmaier, both held all time world records at one time or another and were training partners at the World famous Sampsons Gym in Orange, California.

I began assembling the crew I wanted to training in my garage based upon platform performance and whether they were a great teammate- committed to getting stronger themselves and in supporting everyone in the crew's mission to get stronger- period.

George Pessel was a phenomenal edition. He had been Mr. LA in 83, then trained with Fred Hatfield personally. As Louie Simmons has said repeatedly- there was no greater U.S. lifter or lifting mind than Fred. He totaled elite in 5 weight classes which I think only Louie and Ed Coan have done. George is a great lifter who is still at it competitively to this day. When he trained at Yorba Barbell, he was squatting over 600, benching 500 in training, and pulling over 600 in the 220lb class as a Masters level lifter in his early 40s. George, like most of the other members of Yorba was from South Orange County and had trained together for years prior to training in my garage- which is in northern most Orange County.

Brian Meek had trained with everyone from South Orange County as well, prior to joining the crew at YB. Prior to training at my gym, the spots to train at in South Orange County were Powerhouse Gyms in Lake Forest, Fountain Valley, and Huntington Beach. There were powerlifting monsters such as Hank Hill and Tony Hardridge- world champs who inhabited those gym's at the time. In order to attract a crew to train with me, I would need to be successful, train hard, be a leader, have great equipment and see that everyone who joined the team had the ability to become better due to the phenomenon of a competitive gym environment every workout.

Now don't think we all followed the same exact training protocol when we trained together, because we did not. What we did do was always train the same lift at the same time. Thursday night was heavy bench and Saturday morning was heavy lower body. With my work and long commute, I would do a lighter bench/ shoulder workout on Mondays- or Sunday if I had a ball buster of a work day Monday and I would do dynamic effort squats on Tuesday- often by myself or just with Gary Hogan who lived closest. Most of the members traveled over 20 miles to my garage, which is no easy ride in Southern California traffic.

Rick Purchase was stubborn and did more of a linear periodization workout. Recently, when I posted a picture of Rick, his long time training partner Art LaBare posted that no one worked as hard as Rick in the gym.

Brian Meek was many times National Champion as well as a World Champion Masters level lifter who was over 50 when he joined us but very strong still. Brian was squatting close to 800, benching over 500 and could deadlift over 700. He was enthusiastic to train with, insightful and encouraging. He was the only member of Yorba Barbell who I had been reading about since I was in high school. Brian added so much knowledge, positivity and culture to the crew. One thing that I learned from Brian, was to introduce yourself to every famous lifter you could when you were at a contest or saw them at another gym. Brian introduced me to Gary Frank, Jim Voronin, Mary Ellen Warman, and so many all time greats that I can't remember today. What I do recall and and became a key philosophy of my gym- build allies everywhere you can.

Squat day at Yorba Barbell was Saturday, beginning at 9 am. Since we were all heavyweight 242 lb class and above, it was best for us to squat early on Saturdays so when the contest came around we would be ready to squat at 11 or later- when the heavier classes would have to squat. Squats were done off a set of adjustable hydraulic racks. Due to the fact we were all USPF lifters, we used a Texas power bar for all our three lifts. We did not have a longer, 55lb squat bar even when we transitioned to APF meets in California and at the National level. The only specialty bar was a Crepinsek Safety Squat bar and a Manta Ray device we would snap on to the regular bar.

In the 8 weeks leading up to a contest we would all squat heavy, for a single repetition- adding gear as we got closer to the meet. Once a lifter hit 405 a belt was added, for lifts over 500 or 600lbs squat briefs were added. Squat suits were placed on over briefs and knee wraps were added as well for lifts over 700lbs. Full gear was worn for 800plus pound attempts. Josh Bryant squatted 903, Art Labare did 870, Brian Meek squatted over 800, I did 810, Gary Garcia squatted over 800, Rick did 750, George was over 700 and Gary handled 700 in the squat. We all did not train the same way, but the key was we all squatted heavy and for a single.

I would follow the Westside Barbell system of squatting for a max effort single to a low box- 99% of the time this was a 12" box. I had personal records for this box height with a belt only, with briefs and a belt, with all my gear - suit straps down. After hitting a PR box single, I would do a few sets of power good mornings with either 405 or 500 on the bar for sets of 3 repetitions. This built incredible static strength in my erectors and I never missed a squat due to back strength. I was able to squat 900 in the gym on a few occasions and I attribute the power good morning as being essential for my squat success. Gary Hogan would squat similar to me. Art Labare did box squats with me, but in the offseason. Prior to a meet, he would squat with his gear just as if he was in a contest. Art squatted 850 at my gym and 870 at the inaugural WPO Championships in

Florida. George Pessel and Josh Bryant squatted both ways - free and to boxes at times.

Brian Meek, Rick Purchase, and Gary Garcia never box squatted with us, but they would squat heavy with various stages of supportive gear on. The most important aspect of our squatting philosophy was that we always trained as heavy as possible and we squatted deep. No one from my gym ever bombed out of a meet due to a squat depth issue and we took pride in keeping each other honest when we trained.

After squats we would deadlift, with me and Gary H utilizing the Westside Barbell dynamic percentage cycle of 15 singles at 65%, 12 at 70%, 10 at 75%, 8 at 80%, and 6 singles at 85%. This 5 week cycle worked great for allowing us to pull heavy after a full meet. Art would pull like this in the offseason as did Josh, but Gary G, George, Brian, and Rick did heavy singles in their pulls. Everyone in the gym pulled over 700 officially, with Josh doing 810 and Art at 793 to lead the pack eventually.

We didn't do much assistance work after we squatted heavy, sometimes heavy bent over rows were done. Abdominal work was done heavily and for low repetitions. Floor based Janda sit ups with a partner holding your feet down and weight behind the head made our abs strong.

Thursday was heavy bench night at Yorba and the philosophy was similar to squat day- going heavy was the key. Not everyone followed the Westside method like I did, but Gary H, Gary G. Brian Meek, and George Pessel would do board presses with me- but Art would not. Everyone incline benched and floor pressed in the off season. The last 6 weeks before a meet, bench shirts were used to determine what weights would be smashed at the upcoming meet. On days we would work up to a heavy single in the shirt, after shirt work, we would go raw for sets of 3 in the competition grip as well as the close grip bench. This was a very basic and extremely effective program outlined by Westside Barbell's JM Blakey in a PLUSA Magazine article.

Off season benching involved more repetition work to build muscle and recover from the beating the shoulders and arms took from pre-contest benching and heavy low bar squatting. Art did a very effective and simple program of benching 315 for 5, 10, 15, 20, then go for broke AMRAP. This program resulted in me getting my best ever 315 for 15 raw. I would experiment with reverse grip benching, dumbbell pressing at all angles, and military press work in the offseason with Gary H, but the others would not train like that.

On dynamic effort days for benching and squatting, I would move quickly as the pace on the max efforts days of Thursday and Saturday was not the quickest as we pushed the limits of our strength and added gear and had up to ten lifters at times in my garage as there were times others joined us- but I am only focusing on the core members. For dynamic squats I would follow the Westside three week wave of 50, 55, and 60 percent for 12 to 10 doubles on the box squat of 12" with minimal rest between sets. Heavy bent rows and then abdominal work- like side bends with 150lb dumbbells, would finish the workout.

The dynamic bench workout was 8 triples with 65%, with no accommodating resistance at that time. Shoulder work followed, such as plate raises, Bradford presses, seated dumbbell power cleans, and lateral raises all done quickly and for higher reps. Tricep work was either Dicks presses or tricep extensions with a straight bar or dumbbells. Lat pull downs, one arm rows, hammer curls, and leg raises would round out the day.

One of the key to my lower back health was that I did Dimel deadlifts as Louie prescribed them- 4 times per week I did 2 sets of 20 reps raw with 25% of my deadlift. For a 600lb puller, you would use 135 at the end of each workout. This really conditioned my spine, hamstrings and burned useless fat off my waist. We had no access to a reverse hyper at this time but we found the Dimels kept us all healthy. No one had any back issues ever.

Using this philosophy everyone got strong, everyone became at least a t State and most of us a National champion and we had a blast doing it. Training was always fun, no drudgery here like some gyms had- and few injuries in the actual gym or contests.

If I knew then....

Hindsight is always 20/20, or better. Looking back, what could I have done differently in training, creating a gym, and becoming a better lifter? I am brutally honest when I examine my performance and I won't be shy either in giving myself credit where I did something right.

When I became a competitive powerlifter in 1986, I had a mental focus that was strong for a teenager. I had the ability to realize early on in my strength athlete that I needed to be around stronger people and I always sought those people out. From age 17 onward, I always had a training partner who was stronger than me in a significant way or lift. I was fiercely loyal to my partners and they were with me as well. If I were to go back to my late teen years, I would have broadened my circle some by traveling around more to the various gyms in New England that had amazing powerlifters and bodybuilders in order to learn more. I now realize that I was so fiercely independent, I limited the amount of information and influence I received in my formative strength building years.

In 2022, with the social media connectivity, so many great lifters, coaches, and sources of information to a make yourself a better athlete are at the touch of your fingertip. I have never approached a powerlifter whom I looked up to or wanted to learn from and been turned away or disappointed in my interaction with them. Today, prior to meeting with any great lifter- a person could learn so much about that lifter from their social media and online content- that their interaction should be positive.

Today doctors and medical professionals are more supportive of athletes who are interested in optimal performance while maintaining their long term health. I saw my first chiropractor in Massachusetts when I was 19 and I had badly strained ligaments in my lower back doing exaggerated range of motion stiff leg deadlifts.

He went over an X-ray with me and told me that I had the lower back of a 70 year old. That would mean in 2003 when I pulled my lifetime best of 750- my back was 87 years old. Compare this to my experience with meeting and be treated by the amazing Dr. Joseph Horrigan in Los Angeles.

Dr. Horrigan was a chiropractor who specialized in rotator cuff rehabilitation and wrote for

Ironman Magazine in the 80s and 90s. He loved powerlifters and had treated Dave Shaw, Fred Hatfield and the Barbarian Brothers. Joe fixed my rotator cuff injury as well as my training partner Gary and he taught us how to train our shoulders correctly so that 25 years later, I am still able to press with my shoulders. I have never found another chiropractor as good as Joe- but I have seen therapies on line that you can apply to yourself similarly that are helpful.

Some examples of simple modalities you can do for yourself are on Donnie Thompson's social media, SmashWrx social media and the material Stan Efferding champions such as the ten minute walks after each meal as well as HIT cardio sessions if you want to take off a large amount of powerlifting body weight. I have always loved to walk and have done ao multiple times per day even when I was 325. I would do it instinctively after meals- but if I went back to the 90s, I would have done it after my last big meal of the day before bed.

I once competed in a drug tested Federation against a man who said he was on TRT. He was 26 and bald. I never saw him compete in that federation, so someone was doing their job. In the 90s, it was hard to find a Doctor who would support your need to go on testosterone replacement therapy. They were scarce and expensive. Today, there are doctors everywhere as well as online options if you want to explore TRT or other pharmaceuticals that help you recover to lift more. I, along with some of my Yorba teammates found a great doctor who cared about us and made sure we stayed healthy. I was 30 when I began my treatment. Everyone who I know that worked with this Dr and followed his advice had a long successful career on the platform and most importantly- are all healthy today.

Food choices are easier for lifters today as their are meal preparation services. I am a big fan of everything Stan Efferding so his vertical diet is my style of eating today and I believe he has the best quality meal service in my opinion.

With social media today it is hard not to overtrain with all the inspiring daily posts of huge lifts or meet performances. A lifter today needs to use those influences as fuel for their fire to rest and make progress by sticking to their own programming. I know at my competitive best, I took my scheduled rest days and I did not change from the path of Westside Barbell's program and philosophy. I rested as necessary and because informed came from Westside only once per month via PLUSA, I did not "stray from the way" as Louie says.

If could go back to my beginning, I would have learned to swim better. I love the water and lived on a coast until I was 36, yet I never learned how to really swim well. How would that have helped my lifting? Look at the pressing power of Eddie Hall, James Strickland, Kiril Sarychev, Matt Wenning and James Strickland- all have at least a 612 raw bench and they were all excellent junior level swimmers. Eddie and James were on competition teams for sure. I believe that if I had swam like a competitive swimmer I would have had a much greater bench press and cardio base for my training.

I would have capitalized on my gym if I knew how popular and lucrative gym culture would turn out to be. I modeled my gym after the Westside barbell club model- but none of their business model. I sold only VHS training tapes from my gym at the turn of the millennium, but just enough to buy all the equipment I needed and to pay for any lifting related expenses like travel, food, supplements, therapy, medical care, and supportive gear of the day.

Dr Ken Leistner was a huge influencer in the powerlifting community from the late 1970s until his passing in 2019. Dr Ken promoted my gym and sale of my VHS tape in his

Powerlifting USA Magazine column. If I could go back, I should have started my own website and message board such as Go Heavy and Deepsquatter-which were the premiere powerlifting websites at the turn of the millennium. I had a desire to better the lifters I knew and trained with- but I did not follow the lead of Westside Barbell and create a website that could help so many more.